Contraception

Contraception

The Health Provider's Guide

Cedric W. Porter, M.D., M.P.H.

Obstetrician/Gynecologist
Asheville, North Carolina

Ronald S. Waife, M.S.P.H.

Director of Communications Programs
The Pathfinder Fund
Chestnut Hill, Massachusetts

Hugh R. Holtrop, M.D.

Chief, Department of Obstetrics and Gynecology
San Joaquin General Hospital
Associate Clinical Professor of Obstetrics and Gynecology
University of California, Davis
Stockton, California

Illustrated by E. Penelope Pounder

Grune & Stratton, Inc.
Harcourt Brace Jovanovich, Publishers
Orlando   San Diego   San Francisco   New York   London
Toronto   Montreal   Sydney   Tokyo   São Paulo

Portions of this book have appeared in publications of
The Pathfinder Fund and are used by permission.
All of the illustrations are copyrighted by The Pathfinder Fund
and are used with their permission.
A paperbound edition of this book, which omits Chapter 5
on early abortion techniques and is entitled
The Health Provider's Guide to Contraception,
is available to family planning professionals in
developing countries by writing to The Pathfinder Fund.

Library of Congress Cataloging in Publication Data

Porter, Cedric W.
    Contraception: The health provider's guide.

    Bibliography
    Includes index.
    1. Contraceptives.   I. Waife, Ronald S.   II. Holtrop,
Hugh R.   III. Title.
RG137.P67   1983   613.94'3   83-12857
ISBN 0-8089-1558-4

Grune & Stratton, Inc.
111 Fifth Avenue
New York, New York 10003

Distributed in the United Kingdom by
Grune & Stratton, Inc. (London) Ltd.
24/28 Oval Road, London NW 1

Library of Congress Catalog Number 83-12857
International Standard Book Number 0-8089-1558-4

Printed in the United States of America

To Sarah and to Doug

Contents

Acknowledgments

The authors wish to give special recognition to Marilyn Edmunds, M.S.P.H., and Allison L. Stettner, M.P.H., who drafted significant portions of Chapters 1, 4, and 7 and assisted throughout in the production of this book. Special appreciation also goes to the illustrator of this volume, E. Penelope Pounder, for her educative artistry.

The contraceptive methods that are available today are one of the remarkable achievements of the 20th century. Reliable, safe, and effective means of preventing unwanted birth are so new in mankind's history that their acceptance and use are often hindered by their very newness. Contraception is not yet as basic to human life as are shelter, work, and sex, but it is rapidly becoming so. Family planning—the prevention or spacing of births so that all pregnancies are wanted and are as healthy as possible—has been made a realistic goal by modern contraception. Because of the great contributions to physical and psychological health provided by family planning and because women and men still need guidance, screening, and medical skills to use many of the available contraceptive methods, it is essential that most health providers be thoroughly familiar with contraception. This book is intended to be a comprehensive, concise, and up-to-date guide to the provision of this essential health service.

CHOICES

Choice is a key concept in family planning. While there is no perfect contraceptive method, some methods will be more suitable to a particular client's needs than others. Clients must be offered the full range of methods available in the community, and health providers must help explain how these methods vary in convenience, effectiveness, and appropriateness. *User perspective* and *informed choice* are common phrases in the family planning field that have important meaning—a concern and respect for individual client needs and desires with a nondirective, open approach to contraceptive counseling and education.

Clinical decisions in family planning are often as subjective for the provider as contraceptive choice is for the client. Family planning is a series of choices; there is no one solution, such as using drug A for disease B. The choices that both provider and client must make include: Should contraception be used? To prevent pregnancy or space pregnancies? Which method is most suitable? Which kind of product or technique within each method? When should the method be started? Stopped? Switched? If there is an unplanned pregnancy, should it be continued? If there are side effects, how should they be treated? This book helps the health provider to work with the client in answering most of these questions.

FAMILY PLANNING AND HEALTH

We should remember that family planning is not simply desirable behavior, it is also critically important to physical and psychological well-being. Research has repeatedly shown the physical dangers to mothers and children of having too many pregnancies too soon and too close together. The psychological costs of unwanted pregnancy, to the child and the family as a whole, are also well documented. Family planning is an integral part of improving public welfare, particularly in countries where the pressures of population size and limited resources are great or where maternal and child health conditions are poor. In countries like the United States, family planning has a significant health impact on specific groups such as sexually active adolescents. Thus contraception should be, and is rapidly becoming, a basic part of the general education for all physicians, nurses, and other health personnel.

Health providers need to remember how broad an impact the use of family planning can have on a people's livelihood. At the 1981 International Conference on Family Planning, delegates from more than 90 countries issued the "Jakarta Statement," which included the following words:

> Family planning is an essential component of any broad-based development strategy that seeks to improve the quality of life for both individuals and communities. . . . The lives of millions of mothers and children will be saved [through family planning]. . . . Family planning is a basic human right.

These concepts are hallmarks of our approach to contraceptive practice.

ABOUT THIS BOOK

This book has a unique breadth, and its language is geared to nonspecialist physicians and nonphysicians, including administrators and counselors. We seek to cover all aspects of nonsurgical clinical contraception—counseling, contraceptive mechanisms, contraceptive techniques, management of side effects and complications, and conditions for referral. In addition, the techniques for providing the essential service of pregnancy termination are taught here, with appropriate emphasis on sensitive counseling and postprocedure contraception. Sterilization procedures are discussed in the context of a health provider counseling a client about the sterilization option, but the discussion stops short of surgical instruction.*

This material represents our judgment of the current issues and controversies related to contraceptive practice, a judgment based on our clinical experience and that of others both in the United States and in many developing countries and on our review of literally thousands of articles. Each chapter has a list of selected readings that represent a small fraction of the references surveyed. The listed readings have been chosen because they are classics in the field, represent the latest opinions on controversial topics, or are likely to be most accessible to readers.

One of the unique aspects of family planning practice is that we serve people who usually are not ill or diseased—they are healthy women and men. Thus in this book we use the word *client* to refer to those seeking or using contraception, since they are not patients in the traditional sense of the word. (The only exception is in Chapter 5, where we refer to women undergoing abortion as *patients*.)† People seek guidance and services for family planning in much the same way that they seek lawyers and therapists. Using the terms

---

*Two award-winning training films, produced by The Pathfinder Fund, are available to supplement the material in this text. *Pelvic Examination for Contraception* covers three topics: pelvic examination, intrauterine device insertion, and diaphragm fitting. *Minilaparotomy Techniques* is a training film for surgeons interested in learning the minilaparotomy female sterilization technique referred to in Chapter 6. Information on ordering these films for preview or purchase can be obtained by writing the Communications Programs Department of The Pathfinder Fund, 1330 Boylston Street, Chestnut Hill, Massachusetts 02167.

†We do, however, use feminine pronouns to refer to clients. Although we recognize that some family planning clients are men, and indeed we strongly encourage male participation in contraception, we realize that the majority of clients at this time are women.

provider and *client* will help us remember two critical aspects of family planning practice: many kinds of workers can provide services, and the people we are serving are, for the most part, seeking *preventive* health care—they are healthy and have every right to expect to remain so.

Another of the unique aspects of our practice is the myriad of settings, from hospitals to street corners, in which family planning services are provided all over the world. We use the term *health provider* to mean all of the people working to make contraception available, including physicians, nurses, program administrators, drugstore employees, and community distributors, among many others. From a health point of view, physicians are not required for the provision of many family planning services. This is just as true for the United States as for any developing country, and great savings in health service resources can often be obtained by encouraging nonphysician delivery of family planning wherever possible.

Because most health providers work in a clinical setting, this book focuses on the clinical provision of contraception. As a consequence, certain sections of the text are more technical than others and may require additional explanation for some workers. Our clinical emphasis enables us to discuss contraception more completely than otherwise but in no way represents a bias against nonclinical distribution. In fact, we encourage innovative approaches to family planning services that ensure the widest availability of safe and effective contraception.

We also recognize that some readers may concentrate on only one or two of the chapters, and we thus have written this book in such a way that individual chapters can stand alone. Consequently, some material may seem repetitive. However, *all* health providers delivering contraceptive services should read Chapter 1 on counseling and education closely, since an understanding of client concerns is essential to good practice.

Counseling and Education

Counseling and education are important steps in providing family planning services. More than most health care situations, the provision of contraception involves *choice*. Family planning clients are essentially healthy individuals, and there are few who *must* use one particular method. Counseling and education provide the foundation for the client's choice of contraceptive method and understanding how to provide this foundation is essential for every family planning provider. This chapter, which precedes detailed descriptions of each contraceptive method, reviews the techniques of counseling and education with which every health provider must be familiar.

COUNSELING VERSUS EDUCATION

Unfortunately, many providers fail to distinguish between the terms *counseling* and *education* (Table 1-1). The term *contraceptive counseling* is commonly, yet inaccurately, used to refer to either one. It is true that counseling most often involves education, or at least information-sharing; however, the reverse is not always true: education alone is *not* counseling. Many health workers who provide general information about contraceptive methods do not actually counsel clients, nor should they be expected to do so without the appropriate training. Counseling, by definition, involves helping the client deal with feelings, using specific information-gathering techniques. Education, on the other hand, imparts information

Table 1-1. Counseling Versus Education.
Counseling: helping the client deal with feelings, using specific information-gathering techniques
Education: information given to the client without facilitating decision-making

in an instructive fashion but does not routinely include advice or assistance in decision-making.

Most health professionals agree that family planning clients should learn about contraceptive methods—how they work and possible side-effects. A variety of factors, however, may affect whether the individual providing such information functions primarily as an educator or a counselor and whether the contact is "one-to-one" or in small group sessions. The foremost factor is the provider's background and training. Nurses, social workers, health educators, and community health workers each bring their own frame of reference to the client interaction; some are trained to teach and others, to focus on decision-making. Although the content of information may be similar, individual and professional styles will differ.

Two other factors likely to affect contraceptive education and/or counseling are the client's needs and the clinical setting. It is important to keep in mind that not all family planning clients come to the clinic for the same reason. Some have decided to use contraception and need assistance in choosing a specific method. Others have already decided on the method and seek the clinical care required to implement that decision. Still others come to find out if they are pregnant, and depending on the result, may or may not have a problem to solve. Each of these situations requires a different response.

Clinical settings may also determine the manner in which contraceptive information is provided. In some settings, such as those that serve adolescents, it may be advantageous to have a social worker or other professional *counselor* talk with clients about their contraceptive decisions. In other clinical settings, particularly those in rural areas, community health workers or other *educators* may be found to be more appropriate.

Occasionally there may be a language problem between counselor and client. When the provider does not speak the client's language, counseling cannot occur without an interpreter. If there is no other counselor available who does speak the language in question, either a relative or friend of the client, or another provider who speaks both languages, can interpret.

A different language problem occurs when providers use "jargon" or technical terms that the client does not know. One of the fundamentals of good counseling communication is choosing language that the client can easily understand. When unfamiliar medical terms are used, the counselor must carefully explain their meanings.

Although professional backgrounds and specific clinical roles and responsibilities may differ, it is desirable to establish a baseline knowledge level for individuals providing contraceptive education and counseling. Since a significant number of providers are not professional counselors, some training in basic communication skills and counseling techniques is required.

Depending on the number of clients, clinic facilities, and patient flow patterns, contraceptive education or counseling can be provided in small group sessions. When a clinic is short-staffed or when the clients' background and knowledge are essentially similar, group sessions are particularly helpful. If group sessions are used, however, it is important to conduct them in a large private area of the clinic where clients will feel comfortable asking sensitive questions. Group sessions also give clients the opportunity to learn from the questions and concerns that others raise.

Although group education can help to minimize client waiting time and make efficient use of provider time, an individual interview is vital at some point during the initial visit. For many people, there will be questions that they would hesitate to ask in a group setting but would ask freely in a one-on-one situation.

COUNSELING AND COMMUNICATION TECHNIQUES

Counseling is an on-going process that begins with the exploration and expression of the client's feelings about a particular problem situation. The primary goal of all counseling is to facilitate successful decision-making by reducing anxiety, lending support, providing information regarding alternatives, and assisting in the implementation of the chosen course of action. A good counselor focuses on the circumstances, facts, and feelings that relate to the client's problem. Education, although often an adjunct to some

Table 1-2. Counseling Techniques.
• Establishment of rapport • Expression of empathy • Effective questioning • Active listening • Confrontation of client's feelings • Assistance in decision-making

types of counseling, is not by definition part of the counseling process. As a result of the counseling interaction, the client emerges with increased self-confidence and ability to solve her problem.

Two important fundamentals of a positive counseling interaction are the establishment of rapport and trust and the expression of empathy (Table 1-2). Rapport between counselor and client develops gradually and is by no means automatic. Subtleties of communication such as the counselor's body language, tone of voice, and general manner contribute more to the establishment of trust than does the content of the exchange. To display empathy, the counselor must draw on her own emotional experience to accurately understand the client's feelings while remaining sufficiently detached to differentiate personal feelings from the client's.

Three general techniques integral to all types of counseling are effective questioning, active listening, and confronting feelings. The art of *effective questioning* involves knowing when to ask specific types of questions. At first the counselor should ask open-ended questions that encourage the client to explore her feelings aloud and to focus on *her* thoughts about the problem. "What are your feelings about family planning?" exemplifies the open-ended question. The client cannot answer "yes" or "no" and in most cases will offer information that leads the counselor to further questions. Sometimes the counselor may need to provide the client with some encouragement to talk or short phrases such as "tell me more about . . . " or "go on." This technique often generates additional information that may help to clarify the primary problem at hand. Asking several questions in succession can assist the counselor in gathering information but can also be overwhelming to the client. The counselor must allow time between questions for the client to formulate thoughtful answers.

Leading questions, which limit the range of the response, are useful later in the counseling session. A leading question can either steer the client toward a particular response or help her to focus on a specific area. Questions such as "Do you feel certain that an intrauterine device (IUD) is the best choice for you at this time?" or "Do you think you can comfortably discuss this with your partner now?" are leading questions. This type of questioning summarizes what has gone on in the session and provides the client with direction for her action once the session is over.

Another important counseling technique is *active listening*, which means not only listening to the content of the client's words, but also paying attention to the nonverbal cues she expresses. For example, a woman may appear agitated, even though she denies being nervous, by looking anxiously around the room, playing with her hair, wringing her hands, or similar mannerisms. Other emotions such as anger, mistrust, or depression can be suspected by observing appropriate clues. The counselor should follow this behavioral evidence by encouraging the woman to express any hidden discomforts.

Perhaps the most difficult part of the counseling process involves helping the client *confront* her *feelings* about the problem. First, the counselor must help the client to feel comfortable with her feelings. In order to do this, however, the counselor must assure herself that she has an accurate understanding of the feelings being expressed. During the session the counselor should periodically check her perceptions of what the client is saying ("Do I understand you to mean . . . ?"). Once the counselor understands what the client is feeling, the counselor can confirm the validity of those feelings and help the client to accept them. Confronting feelings will reduce anxiety and allow for more productive decision-making.

The four most common emotions that surface during counseling are guilt, fear, ambivalence, and anger. The first two—guilt and fear—need to be overcome at the beginning to make the client feel comfortable with considering family planning in the first place. Once the decision-making stage is reached, ambivalence and anger become the primary obstacles.

Guilt is an emotion commonly expressed in family planning counseling. The counselor's task is to find out why the client feels guilty and then help the client put those feelings in perspective. For instance, the client may have been told by her family or religion that it is "wrong" to prevent conception. Such guilt can be diminished if the client realizes that her true feelings do not match those of outside influences. Resolution of guilt feelings is a key step in preparing the client for a contraceptive choice.

Clients are also often fearful of the clinical procedures that they may encounter during their visit. Some people have a generalized fear of physicians and health care, whereas others have more specific fears relating to pain and illness. During the counseling session, time should be taken to identify these fears and discuss them. If a client does not mention being afraid, the counselor should anticipate the possibility of unexpressed fear and provide an opportunity for talking about it.

Once the client feels comfortable with considering family planning, ambivalence and anger will be common obstacles to reaching a final contraceptive choice. The term *ambivalence* refers to having conflicting emotions about a particular situation. Family planning clients often feel ambivalent about many aspects of their clinic visit—whether or not to use contraception, which method to use, whether or not they are pregnant, or whether or not to undergo surgery. It is important to stress to the client that such ambivalence is natural and then help her to evaluate her feelings both pro and con before making a final decision. Coming to terms with ambivalent feelings can be time-consuming and may comprise a major portion of the counseling session. Although care must be taken to avoid rushing the client, it may sometimes be necessary to direct her toward a decision as the session closes. In no instance should a decision be forced on the client, but in some cases a follow-up session may need to be scheduled to allow ample time for the ambivalence to be resolved.

Family planning clients often express anger during the counseling session. A woman may be angry about the process involved in obtaining contraception. She may be angry about the limited options open to her specific situation. Or she may be angry with her partner, particularly if he assumes little responsibility for birth control or does not support her visit to the clinic. In such cases anger often protects the woman from feeling vulnerable, providing a defense against her insecurities. The counselor can help the woman to understand and accept her vulnerability. It is important, too, for the woman to recognize that anger in this situation is not unusual; the energy generated can be used to take constructive action toward her family planning decision.

Above all, an effective counselor provides nonjudgmental support to the client during the decision-making process by showing empathy, giving information, clarifying feelings, and outlining alternative actions. Other responsibilities will vary depending on both the type of counseling and the setting in which it occurs.

CONTRACEPTIVE EDUCATION

Contraceptive education often begins before the client attends the information session. Waiting areas can be designed with attractive posters outlining the various contraceptive methods. Pamphlets and brochures describing health benefits of family planning and other aspects of contraceptive use can be placed throughout the clinic for clients to read. Contraceptive education materials will often help a client to focus on specific questions or concerns she wants to have addressed during her visit. If at all possible, such materials should be designed for clients to take with them for future reference and should include information on how to contact the provider.

Health workers providing contraceptive education and/or counseling should be knowledgeable about the technical aspects of contraception. Having a background in one of the health or allied professions is not essential but can be advantageous. Training programs for providers must be comprehensive and cover a broad range of topics, including male and female reproductive anatomy and physiology, contraceptive methods and how they work (including abortion and sterilization procedures), contraindications and side-effects, the effectiveness rates of different methods, psychosocial aspects of human sexuality, and any additional information relevant to the specific client group being served. Educators should be able to communicate general information to new family planning clients and also to discuss more specific issues and concerns with returning clients. The general training requirements for educators are listed in Table 1-3.

Contraceptive educators should clearly explain the menstrual cycle and describe hormonal changes that allow pregnancy to occur. The male reproductive cycle should also be discussed, outlining the stages from sperm production to sperm transport and ejaculation.

Table 1-3.
Training Requirements for Educators.

- Male–female reproductive anatomy and physiology
- Contraceptive methods and how they work
- Contraindications and side-effects
- Psychosocial aspects of human sexuality
- Basic communication skills for individuals and groups

Once the client understands both the menstrual cycle and the male reproductive cycle, she can more readily comprehend various contraceptive methods and their function.

Specific method-related information is reviewed in Chapters 2–4; abortion and sterilization procedures are discussed in Chapters 5 and 6. Contraceptive educators should learn the information given in these chapters and adapt the presentation to their clients. Family planning clients must receive complete yet concise information about all available methods in order to make an appropriate contraceptive decision.

In helping clients to make contraceptive decisions, family planning providers may inadvertently imply that the choice of method is a final one. Although the goal of counseling is for the client to identify the method she thinks will best suit her individual situation, the possibility of method-switching should not be excluded from the discussion. A woman may try one method for a while but experience bothersome side-effects or simply discover that it is not as convenient to use as she had thought. Counselors should anticipate these occurrences and reassure the client that she can return at any time to obtain a different method. Many providers tend to consider a high frequency of method-switching as undesirable. But they should recognize that method-switching at least means that the client is highly motivated to use contraception, which is distinct from those clients who discontinue contraceptive use altogether. It should be emphasized, however, that the risk of unwanted pregnancy increases during the time when the contraceptive method is changed. Therefore, clients should be encouraged to overlap two methods to avoid any period when contraception is not used.

Contraindications, Side-Effects, and Effectiveness Rates

A thorough explanation of contraception includes more than how individual methods work. Potential contraindications—physical conditions that should preclude a woman's use of a particular method—and possible side-effects often affect a client's method selection, as does the method's effectiveness at preventing pregnancy. Providers should assist the client in using this information to compare methods according to her individual needs.

Major and minor side-effects associated with each method should be clearly explained. It is important to differentiate between commonly held beliefs and carefully documented research data. Yet

Table 1-4.
Theoretical Versus Use Effectiveness.
Theoretical effectiveness: an effectiveness rate that could be achieved *if* the method is *always* used correctly
Use effectiveness: an effectiveness rate that reflects actual practice if a couple is as successful as average users

it is also a mistake to belittle potential side-effects in an attempt to encourage method acceptance. If a client experiences unanticipated nausea or breakthrough bleeding with the pill, for example, she may think something is wrong and discontinue use, whereas if these side-effects had been explained to her beforehand, she would understand that they usually pass within the first few months. The risk of more serious complications associated with each method should be neither exaggerated nor minimized. Accurate presentation of these risks in their proper perspective is a challenge that every counselor-educator must study carefully. Frank discussion of side-effects that commonly occur, as well as those experienced less frequently, will be beneficial to both the client and the clinician.

Clients should determine an acceptable level of method effectiveness for their current situation and then compare effectiveness rates for available methods. The most objective way to present comparative effectiveness rates is to give two rates for each method: (1) the level of effectiveness that would be achieved if the couple used the method perfectly all the time, or *theoretical effectiveness;* and (2) the level of effectiveness to be expected if the couple is as successful as "average" users, or *use effectiveness* (Table 1-4). Effectiveness rates give only a general idea of how well other people have used a method in the past; each couple determines a method's effectiveness by their care and consistency in its use. It is important to point out, too, that combining barrier methods (e.g., condoms and foam) can dramatically improve effectiveness.

Good counseling and education, when provided together, will help each other: contraceptive information can help in decision-making, and confronting feelings can help the client in proper method use. Psychological as well as physiological aspects of human sexuality contribute to the acceptance and effectiveness of contraception. A skilled provider can help the client to improve her contraceptive decision-making by providing accurate information about sexuality and sexual behavior. When discussing these topics, the provider must be especially mindful of sociocultural factors such as community beliefs and ethical codes that might affect family planning acceptance, and thus effectiveness. It is often advantageous, therefore, that the provider be a community member who shares the clients' cultural traditions and norms.

Social and emotional factors might interfere with the effective use of a particular method. Many variables, including family and peer relationships, educational background, and religious upbringing influence a prospective client's attitudes toward different contraceptive methods. The counseling session will offer a client the chance to express reservations she may have about a particular method that could prevent her from using it regularly, or at all. Bringing these problems into the open may eliminate them as obstacles to successful contraception.

IMPLICATIONS OF FAMILY PLANNING ADOPTION

Reproductive capacity generally contributes to the self-identity of both men and women. The choice to use contraception affects the client, her partner, and the community at large. A woman's place in society may even be defined solely by her ability to conceive and bear children. Men may feel the need to prove their virility by impregnating their partner at regular intervals. Although benefits of contraceptive use may be self-evident to providers, clients may not be aware or convinced of the advantages to practicing family planning.

During the counseling-education process, the provider should explain family planning benefits in a manner that the client can understand and readily apply to her own situation. Both mother and child will enjoy better health when pregnancies are planned and well spaced. Family planning will enable the woman to seek activity and roles outside the home. Time otherwise spent caring for children can be used to acquire new skills and thereby contribute to the woman's personal growth, as well as to the family's income and welfare.

Most family planning methods involve women more directly than men; however, contraceptive effectiveness depends on both partners. Men frequently express reluctance to use condoms, for instance, and some do not want their partners to use contraception either. Reasons for such hesitation vary. In some cultures, family status relates to the number of children. Sometimes a man may strongly desire a male child and may not want to use contraception until a son is born. There may be concern about changes in traditional roles, which sometimes occur when couples use contraception. If a woman is concerned about her partner's acceptance of family planning, the counselor might schedule a joint session to help the couple discuss their feelings openly.

It is the counselor's responsibility to clearly delineate the advantages and disadvantages, risks, and relative merits of all contraceptive methods available. Comprehensive method explanation at the outset will improve the client's ability to make a truly "informed choice." The counseling-education session should encourage the client to think in terms of contraceptive *alternatives.* Too often new contraceptive clients view their method choice as an irrevocable decision. It is important for the client to try to make the most appropriate method choice initially; however, she should understand that other options exist in the event that the first choice does not work out. The provider should remember to emphasize, however, the increased risk of pregnancy that accompanies method-switching, particularly when the woman changes from a method requiring relatively little client participation, such as the IUD, to a more complicated method such as the diaphragm.

FOLLOW-UP AND REFERRAL

When the discussion of technical information has been completed, the provider should briefly summarize what has gone on in the session, giving the client a chance to ask any final questions. To ensure continued safe and effective method use, a follow-up plan must be arranged.

Depending on the clinical setting and the method chosen, follow-up visit intervals will vary. In rural clinics or regions where community-based nonclinical services are available, the follow-up visit may occur in the client's community or even in her home. Clinical methods such as an IUD or diaphragm require a medical follow-up, which simultaneously offers the client another chance to talk with the counselor. Follow-up sessions should be used to help allay fears or hesitation, review method instructions, and encourage regular contact with the health service. The client's work schedule, her responsibilities at home, and possible transportation problems should be considered when setting up return appointments.

Referral is an important aspect of comprehensive family planning care. Both the clinician and the counselor-educator should be prepared to make referrals for other health and social services as needed. Examples of health problems often discovered during a family planning visit include breast lumps, abnormal Papanicolaou (Pap) smears, sexually transmitted disease or other vaginal or ure-thral infections, hypertension, anemia, nutritional deficiencies, and anxiety or depression (see Chapter 7).

When referral is indicated, the nature of the problem should be carefully explained to the patient. If a preexisting health concern affects the client's choice of a family planning method, further coun-seling will be necessary. Whenever possible, the client should be provided with alternative choices for referral services, keeping in mind factors such as accessibility and cost. One should avoid refer-ring clients to unfamiliar resources, unless there is no other option. If clients have been dissatisfied with a referral, the provider should investigate the problem before continuing to use that resource.

Even if no other health problems are identified, the client should know where to go for emergency care. During times when the clinic is closed, the client needs to know to whom to turn in the event of contraceptive-related complications. She should be sup-plied with a description of specific symptoms that may signal com-plications and the need for medical attention.

PREGNANCY COUNSELING

The initial contact between health provider and family plan-ning client is often due to pregnancy—confirmed or unconfirmed, wanted or unwanted. The first step is usually a laboratory test and/or pelvic examination to determine whether the woman is pregnant, followed by a private counseling session to discuss the reliability and implications of the results. The counselor will confront one of two situations—a woman who wants to be pregnant or a woman who does not.

When the client wants to be pregnant and test results are posi-tive, the counselor should discuss early prenatal precautions and make the appropriate medical referral for care throughout the pregnancy.

Abortion is an alternative for most women confronting an un-wanted pregnancy. Counseling should always be an integral part of this service. Most facilities that offer abortion counsel clients both before and after the procedure, but it is important for providers at

Table 1-5.
Steps in Problem Pregnancy Counseling.
• Report pregnancy test results in person • Encourage client to express feelings about the results • Outline available alternatives • Explain means for implementing client's choice • Encourage postpregnancy contraceptive use • Involve the client's partner whenever possible

the family planning clinic to begin emotional support and guidance for the client at the moment of the positive pregnancy diagnosis.

The basic aim of problem pregnancy counseling is to help the woman identify her feelings and make a decision about pregnancy resolution. The counselor then helps the client to implement that decision and to consider options for controlling her future fertility. Equally important, the counselor seeks to ensure that if pregnancy termination is desired, it is accomplished as early as possible to minimize both physical and emotional trauma.

Problem pregnancy counseling ideally consists of several steps (Table 1-5). Initially, the counselor reports test results and helps the woman to express and evaluate her feelings. Next, after alternatives are explored and a choice is made, the counselor explains the procedure to be followed. If the pregnancy is terminated, the counselor should talk with the woman again after the abortion. At this time contraceptive methods should be presented and the counselor should encourage the client to choose a method without delay. Ideally, problem pregnancy counseling should involve the woman's sexual partner as well. This provides a special opportunity for family planning contact with the male. In addition, his active support of the woman's decision can be a critical factor in her resolution of the emotional conflict presented by an unwanted pregnancy. (For more information on pregnancy termination, see Chapter 5.)

CONTRACEPTIVE COUNSELING FOR ADOLESCENTS

Harmful health and social consequences resulting from teenage childbearing are well documented. For the adolescent woman, the risk of the following pregnancy complications is increased: toxemia of pregnancy, stillbirth, neonatal mortality, prematurity, and serious physical or mental handicaps. Early childbearing also commonly leads to having additional children at shorter intervals, which further compromises maternal and infant health. The provision of complete family planning counseling can make an important contribution to adolescents' future health by preventing early pregnancy and spacing future pregnancies.

Reluctance to provide family planning counseling and services to unmarried adolescents stems from several erroneous yet commonly held beliefs. People often fear that providing family planning services to adolescents not only implies tacit acceptance of premarital sexual activity, but actually encourages "promiscuity" by reducing the fear of pregnancy. Available evidence does not, however, support these views. On the contrary, statistics document increased social problems as well as the health risks outlined above for sexually active adolescents who do not use contraception. Family planning services with thorough, sensitive counseling are therefore a public health imperative.

Beyond the usual counseling and educational services already discussed, providers have an additional responsibility to the adolescent seeking contraceptive advice. Teenagers desperately need facts about sexuality to help them overcome the misinformation they often have. They also need more guidance than older clients—more encouragement to help them make their own decisions and take responsibility for their actions. This may be the adolescent's first open discussion of sex, sexuality, and contraception. Quite possibly, it will also be her first pelvic examination. The counselor or educator should anticipate the adolescent client's anxiety, confusion, and uncertainty relating to these new physical and emotional experiences and should acknowledge and respond to those concerns.

First, the counselor should establish whether the adolescent is a willing partner in sexual activity. If the client is feeling pressured, the provider can give her the confidence and support to "say no." Conversely, if the client is comfortable with her role as a sexually active person, this should be accepted in a nonjudgmental fashion. Since both peer pressures and family interactions strongly affect adolescents' decision-making, involvement of the parents and/or the partner can be beneficial if appropriate.

In counseling young clients, special attention should be paid to their immediate contraceptive needs when weighed against any possible long-term effects on health and fertility. The risks associated with each method must also be compared with the high pregnancy risks for adolescents. Family planning counseling for the young cli-

Table 1-6.
Adolescents: Contraceptive Alternatives.

	Advantages	Disadvantages
Condoms	• Readily available without prescription • Decreases risk of sexually-transmitted diseases • Involves the male	• Less effective • Depends on male
Diaphragm	• Lack of systemic effects • Appropriate when intercourse occurs infrequently	• Requires conscientious use and preplanning for effectiveness • Requires touching genitals • Requires prescription
Oral contraceptives	• Effective • Unrelated to intercourse	• May be inappropriate if woman is anovulatory • Must remember to take daily • Requires prescription
IUDs	*If necessary to use:* • Effective • Unrelated to intercourse	• Contraindicated in nulliparas because of increased risk of pelvic inflammatory disease and possibility of subsequent infertility • Requires prescription

ent is not complete without a detailed discussion of sexually transmitted diseases.

Each contraceptive method has special advantages and disadvantages for adolescents (Table 1-6). The condom, for instance, has many advantages for the young couple: it is safe and readily available without need for medical examination or prescription, helps to promote male contraceptive responsibility, and decreases the incidence of sexually transmitted diseases. Although the condom is reasonably effective when used alone, its use effectiveness increases significantly when it is used in combination with contraceptive foam (see Chapter 4).

The diaphragm with spermicidal cream or jelly can offer adolescent users some advantages. Like the condom, a diaphragm is appealing for its lack of systemic effects. It can be particularly appropriate for adolescents who have infrequent intercourse and need contraceptive protection on limited occasions (see Chapter 4). If intercourse is unpredictable as well as infrequent, however, the advance planning necessary for effective diaphragm use may be difficult. In addition, effective diaphragm use is impossible unless the woman is comfortable with manipulation of her genitals. This is sometimes difficult to achieve in adolescents.

Oral contraceptive use by adolescents must be carefully evaluated on the basis of several factors. Many clinicians question the wisdom of prescribing oral contraception to users who may be experiencing anovulatory menstrual cycles. Since younger adolescents often exhibit signs of anovulation in the first postmenarche years, they may not be good candidates for pill use. As with any oral contraceptive user, the counselor should explain to adolescents the risks and benefits of pill use and stress the importance of regular pill-taking and the use of a back-up method if pills are skipped or not taken daily (see Chapter 2).

Intrauterine devices are generally considered undesirable for adolescent use because of their association with increased pelvic infection rates. Since most adolescent clients are nulliparas, the small but possible risk of infertility developing from pelvic infection warrants great caution when considering IUD use in the younger client (see Chapter 3). On the occasions when IUD use might be appropriate for an adolescent, these risks must be explained thoroughly.

On completion of the counseling session, the adolescent client should be able to think clearly about contraceptive options in terms of her specific needs. On the basis of the characteristics of each method, the adolescent should be able to identify the method most compatible with her medical history and sexual habits. The counselor should make it clear to adolescent clients that although there is no ideal contraceptive available, use of any method is better than none. Younger clients in particular need to realize that their initial contraceptive decision is not irrevocable; switching to a different method at a future point is usually an option. They should be informed of the increased risk of pregnancy during the time period surrounding a method change, however, and strongly encouraged to overlap two methods rather than stopping use of one before starting use of another.

A specific follow-up plan should be outlined for each adolescent client. In addition to stressing the importance of clinical follow-up, the client should be encouraged to seek further counseling at the return visit should she have questions or concerns about method use. A successful counseling experience with the adolescent can contribute to responsible contraceptive use throughout the reproductive years.

Often adolescents do not routinely seek medical care. Young persons' visits to a family planning clinic may provide their only access to a medical facility. Counselors should recognize this possibility and be aware of other health needs and problems that frequently face adolescents—accidents, drug and alcohol abuse, developmental difficulties, nutrition, smoking, and sexually transmitted diseases. In some cases it may be necessary to refer the adolescent client to another provider.

Pregnant adolescents require even more specialized counseling services than do adolescents in general. Not only do they face two maturational crises—puberty and pregnancy—simultaneously, they also are in the process of establishing autonomy from their parents. With inadequately developed emotional mechanisms, pregnant adolescents are likely to be under tremendous pressure. Counselors must recognize the importance of parental influence on the emotional health of the adolescent. Parental attitudes will affect guilt, anxiety, and the client's ability to accept contraception in the future. This influence is compounded by the parents' legal and economic control over their child. Considering that during and after pregnancy resolution the family and its attitudes continue to surround the adolescent, the client's confidence in her own decision is critical.

In this situation the counselor faces a delicate task that requires considerable expertise. The counselor must not only assist the adolescent in reaching a decision about pregnancy resolution, but must also help the young client deal with parental reactions to that decision. The provider should guard against getting caught in the middle of a parent–child conflict but can also act as an effective liaison between them.

CONCLUSION

Good communication skills and comprehensive technical information are two important elements of family planning counseling and education. The manner and tone in which family planning communication occurs is the third critical factor. Providers must be comfortable with their own sexuality and be able to consistently convey that message. The counselor-educator's comfort with the subject matter is expressed through body language, ease in use of correct terminology, and the willingness to initiate difficult conversation topics. Although it is not important for providers and clients to share the same values regarding family planning, it is imperative that counselor-educators refrain from imposing their own standards on the client; they must continually demonstrate the ability to be nonjudgmental. Clients must reach their own decisions about contraception if they are to successfully incorporate family planning into their lives.

Selected Readings

Barwin N: Psychological factors: Counseling and motivation of the contraceptive patient. International Journal of Gynecology and Obstetrics 16(6): 568, 1979

Beresford T: Short-Term Relationship Counseling. Baltimore, Planned Parenthood of Maryland, 1977

Bracken MB: Psychosomatic aspects of abortion: Implications for counseling. Journal of Reproductive Medicine 19(5): 265, November 1977

Burchell RC: Counseling in gynecologic practice: an overview. Clinical Obstetrics and Gynecology 21(1): 165, March 1978

Chung KK, Kabar DN, Santiago CE, et al: User preference for contraceptive methods in India, Korea, the Phillipines and Turkey. Studies in Family Planning 11(9/10): 267, September/October, 1980

Cooperman C, Weinstein SA: Contraceptive counselor's dilemma: Safety or effectiveness? The Journal of Sex Research 14(3): 145, August 1978

Diamond M: Contraceptive counseling for sexually active adolescents. Medical Aspects of Human Sexuality 11: 73, November 1977

Dunlop JL: Counseling of patients requesting an abortion. Practitioner 220(1320): 847, June 1978

Ford CV: Psychological factors influencing the choice of contraceptive method. Medical Aspects of Human Sexuality 12(1): 91, January 1978

Freeman EW, Rickels K, Huggins GR, et al: Emotional distress patterns among women having first or repeat abortions. Obstetrics and Gynecology 55(5): 630, May 1980

Gavin J: Selecting the optimum method of contraception for each patient. International Journal of Gynecology and Obstetrics 16(6): 542, 1979

Huggins GR: Counseling patients for contraception. Clinical Obstetrics and Gynecology 22(2): 509, June 1979

Jones EF, Paul L, Westoff, CF: Contraceptive efficacy: The significance of method and motivation. Studies in Family Planning 11(2): 39, February 1980

Kinch RA: The patient's choice in contraception. International Journal of Gynecology and Obstetrics 16(6): 561, 1979

Marcus RJ: Evaluating abortion counseling. Dimensions in Health Service 56(8): 16, August 1979

Mwaniki MK: Perceptions and psychological behaviors toward contraception, in Mwaniki N, Marasha M, Mati JKG, et al: Surgical Contraception in Sub-Saharan Africa (proceedings of a conference, Nyeri, Kenya, May 8–13, 1977). Chestnut Hill, MA, The Pathfinder Fund, 1979

Nadelson CC: Abortion counseling: Focus on adolescent pregnancy. Pediatrics 54(1):6, July 1974

Nadelson CC, Notman MT, Gillon JW: Sexual knowledge and attitudes of adolescents: Relationship to contraceptive use. Obstetrics and Gynecology 55(3): 340, March 1980

Ogden C: Adolescent Fertility: Selected, Annotated Resources for the International Community. Washington, DC, International Clearinghouse on Adolescent Fertility, 1978

Reading AE, Newton JR: Psychological factors in IUD use—a review. Journal of Biosocial Science 9(3): 317, July 1977

Rozenbaum H: Teenagers and contraception. International Journal of Gynecology and Obstetrics 16(6): 564, 1979

Segal SJ: Contraceptives and the young: Present status and future prospects. Pediatrics 62(6) Pt. 2: 1211, December 1978

Spellacy N: Contraception for the high-risk woman. Contemporary Obstetrics and Gynecology 14: 119, August 1979

Vessey M, Doll R, Peto R, et al: A long-term follow-up study of women using different methods of contraception—an interim report. Journal of Biosocial Science 8(4): 375, October 1976

Vessey M, Meisler L, Flavel R, et al: Outcome of pregnancy in women using different methods of contraception. Obstetrical and Gynecological Survey 35(4): 206, April 1980

Zabin LS, Clark SD: Why they delay: A study of teenage family planning clinic patients. Family Planning Perspectives 13(5): 205, September/October 1981

Zeidenstein G: The user perspective: An evolutionary step in contraceptive service programs. Studies in Family Planning 11(1): 24, January 1980

Oral Contraceptives

Oral contraceptives—widely known as "the pill"—have revolutionized family planning since their introduction in 1960. Oral contraceptives have become the most popular fertility control method in many countries and are now being utilized by an estimated 50 million women around the world in a variety of countries and cultures. The contraceptive pill has merited this extensive acceptance: it is the most effective reversible form of contraception, and yet it is safe and convenient. Moreover, oral contraceptives may be safely supplied to most family planning users by well-trained nonphysicians as well as physicians, and in nonclinical as well as clinical settings.

The popularity of oral contraceptives can partly be explained by comparing them with other reversible means of contraception. Consistent pill users can obtain a remarkable effectiveness of contraception close to 99%, which is higher than that of the pill's major alternatives (Figure 2-1). For instance, data from a large-scale retrospective British study by the Royal College of General Practitioners (RCGP), involving 23,000 pill users and 23,000 nonusers followed since 1968, have demonstrated that the pregnancy rate for women continuing to use the pill is 0.34 per 100 woman-years.

After decades of research and literally hundreds of studies, oral contraceptives are among the most intensely studied drugs in history. The results of the largest and longest-running studies have recently shown that the pill's superior effectiveness is achieved with almost complete safety for women under 35 years of age and who do not smoke cigarettes (see page 55). Any risks of oral contraceptive use also must be weighed against the significant health hazards of

21

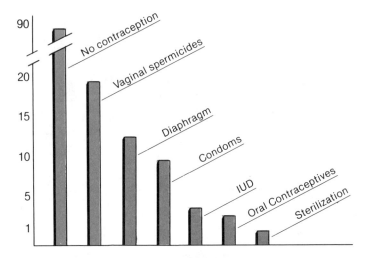

Figure 2-1. *Comparative contraceptive effectiveness, showing range of reported pregnancy rates per 100 woman-years of method use. (Adapted from Vessey et al., 1982, and others.)*

pregnancy—especially in those areas where the maternal mortality rates are high (see Figure 2-11). The risk of death from oral contraceptive use is far less than the risk of mortality from pregnancy itself for most groups of women.

While in past years, every month seemed to bring news of a possible pill-associated health hazard, now new health *benefits* from oral contraceptives are being reported frequently (see page 27). Nevertheless, much attention remains focused on the side-effects and complications of oral contraceptives. Perhaps this is justifiable considering the huge numbers of women taking these drugs for what has always been assumed to be a "secondary" purpose—preventive rather than therapeutic. This assumption is misleading. Pregnancy involves serious health risks; *unwanted* pregnancy adds serious psychosocial risks. Preventing unwanted pregnancy is therefore an important health goal. Any disadvantages of oral contraceptive use should be evaluated from this perspective.

TYPES OF PILLS

Numerous oral contraceptive preparations are available today, the result of an increasing variety of chemical combinations and product names. In general, the types of contraceptive pills break down into two groupings: combined and progestin-only preparations (a progestin is any synthetic hormone with progestational characteristics).

Combined pills. Each of these pills contains two synthetic hormones—an estrogen and a progestin. Combined pills are generally available in standard and low-dose formulas. The combined pill benefits from the contraceptive effects of both hormones and is almost totally effective in preventing pregnancy when taken properly. These preparations are the subject of this chapter.

Progestin-only pills (minipills). These preparations contain small doses of synthetic progestins and obtain their contraceptive effect primarily by altering the cervical mucus (secretion at the neck of the womb), making it inhospitable to sperm transport, and by altering the endometrial environment (lining of the womb), thus inhibiting the implantation of the fertilized egg. Ovulation is not necessarily inhibited by these pills. Minipills are 96%–98% effective in preventing pregnancy an effective rate comparable to the IUD) but are frequently associated with irregular menstrual bleeding and amenorrhea (absence of menstruation). They may be useful in women who have been experiencing estrogen-related problems on other oral contraceptive preparations. Some clinicians use these pills for contraception in lactating mothers, although usually only if no other contraceptive method is suitable and prevention of pregnancy is imperative. Because of the limited clinical applicability of minipills, we do not discuss them further in this publication.

Worldwide, the most frequently used oral contraceptives are the combined pills. This guide highlights two combined preparations: 1 mg of norethindrone (a progestin) with 0.05 mg (50 μg) of mestranol (an estrogen) and 0.5 mg of norethindrone with 0.035 mg (35 μg) of ethinyl estradiol (another estrogen) (Table 2-1). These formulations are representative of the two standard dosages currently available and thus are used to simplify the discussion. It is not meant to imply that these pills are superior to other similar preparations.

Table 2-1. Representative Pill Types	
The 1/50 pill	1 mg norethindrone + 50 μg mestranol
The "low-dose" pill	0.5 mg norethindrone + 35 μg ethinyl estradiol

PHYSIOLOGY

The precise mechanism of the contraceptive effect of oral contraceptives is now generally known after years of exhaustive research. It is believed that the combined oral contraceptive acts by interfering with the normal menstrual cycle in several different ways. A knowledge of the normal cycle is necessary to understand these contraceptive effects.

The first day of menstruation is counted as the beginning of the cycle. Menstruation is the shedding of the endometrium (lining) of the uterus (womb). This occurs if fertilization and implantation of an ovum (egg) have not occurred in the previous cycle. Early in the cycle, the pituitary gland (the "master gland" located at the base of the brain) is stimulated to produce follicle-stimulating hormone (FSH). This substance in turn causes growth of a follicle (sac) in the ovaries that contains the ovum. Estrogen is produced by the maturing ovarian follicle, which stimulates growth of the endometrium. The endometrium becomes thicker and develops a spongelike surface. This is called the *proliferative phase* of the menstrual cycle (Figure 2-2A).

Meanwhile, the rising level of circulating estrogen produced by the ovary begins to inhibit the production of pituitary FSH, the same substance that had stimulated the estrogen production in the first place. This is called a *feedback mechanism* (Figure 2-3). Also during this time, luteinizing hormone (LH) has been building up in the pituitary gland. As FSH decreases, the pituitary gland is stimulated to release its stored LH in a sudden surge. This peak in LH levels is the immediate cause of ovulation (the ovum leaving the follicle in preparation for possible conception).

After ovulation has occurred, the remaining cells from the ovarian follicle form the corpus luteum, a body that produces both estrogen and progesterone. During this time the endometrial surface begins to secrete a mucuslike fluid and the endometrium itself becomes edematous (water-filled) and ceases to grow. This is called the *secretory phase* of the menstrual cycle.

If fertilization does not occur, the corpus luteum shrinks and estrogen and progesterone levels decline so that the endometrium degenerates and menstruation occurs (Figure 2-2A). This takes place approximately 14 days after ovulation. If, on the other hand, the ovum is fertilized and becomes implanted in the endometrium, no menstruation occurs. The corpus luteum continues to produce estro-

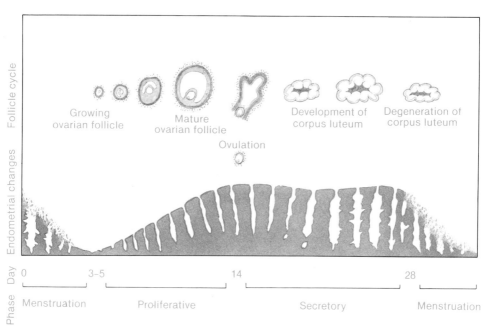

Figure 2-2A. *The normal nonpregnant menstrual cycle.*

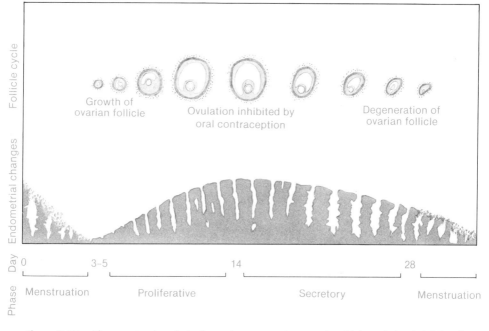

Figure 2-2B. *The menstrual cycle in the oral contraceptive user, in which ovulation is inhibited.*

25

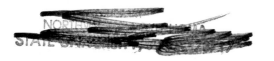

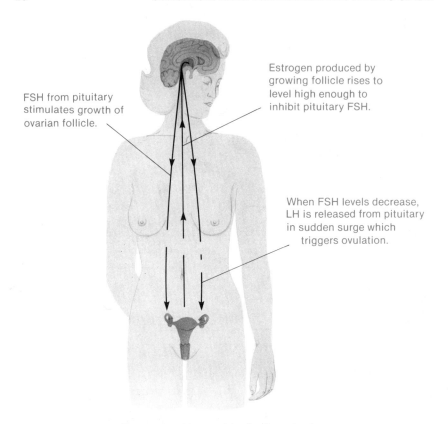

FSH from pituitary
stimulates growth of
ovarian follicle.

Estrogen produced by
growing follicle rises to
level high enough to
inhibit pituitary FSH.

When FSH levels decrease,
LH is released from pituitary
in sudden surge which
triggers ovulation.

Figure 2-3. *Hormonal feedback mechanism.*

gen and progesterone until the developing placenta can provide a
sufficient level of hormones to maintain the pregnancy.

CONTRACEPTION AND
OTHER BENEFICIAL EFFECTS

Combined oral contraceptives are thought to inhibit ovulation
by blocking the production and release of FSH and LH. The estrogenic component of the pill suppresses FSH production, thus preventing ovum development (Figure 2-2B). Both the estrogens and
progestins in these pills appear to inhibit ovulation by blocking the
LH surge.

The combined oral preparations also exert important direct contraceptive effects on the cervical mucus and endometrium. The cervical mucus in women using the combined pill is scanty and dense with tight cellular alignment, providing a physical barrier that blocks passage of spermatozoa into the uterus. The endometrium is also rendered unfavorable to ovum implantation through the combined effects of estrogen and progestin, making the lining more thin and inhospitable than in the normal untreated cycle. Both of the above mechanisms serve to reduce the possibility of pregnancy if ovulation should occur.

In addition to their contraceptive effect, oral contraceptives may have other beneficial effects on the following conditions in certain women (see also Table 2-2):

Dysmenorrhea (menstrual pain). Pills usually minimize menstrual cramps and hence may help to reduce painful menstruation in women so afflicted.

Irregular bleeding. Pills ordinarily produce regular menstrual periods and may be used for symptomatic control of bleeding patterns.

Menorrhagia (heavy menstruation). Pills generally reduce the number of days of menstrual flow. The total amount of blood loss and the intensity of flow during menstruation is also often reduced in oral contraceptive users.

Table 2-2. Conditions Alleviated or Protected Against by Use of Oral Contraceptives.		
Dysmenorrhea	Pelvic inflammatory disease	600*
Irregular bleeding	Iron-deficiency anemia	320
Menorrhagia	Benign breast tumors	235
Mittelschmerz	Ectopic pregnancy	117
Endometriosis	Ovarian cysts	35
	Arthritis	32
	Endometrial cancer	5
	Ovarian cancer	4

Adapted from Kols et al., 1982.
*Number indicates estimate of hospitalizations or disease episodes prevented among 100,000 pill users per year (United States).

Recurrent ovarian cysts and ovarian cancer. Because of the suppression of ovarian activity by oral contraceptives, there is a decreased incidence of functional ovarian cysts in pill users. Data from several studies, including those by the U.S. Centers for Disease Control (CDC) and the RCGP, indicate that the pill's suppression of ovulation also protects against the development of ovarian cancer. The protective effect against this rare but usually fatal condition apparently persists long after cessation of pill use and is particularly pronounced in former pill users over 40 years old.

Therapeutic suppression of ovulation. Oral contraceptives can be used to eliminate ovulatory pain (*mittelschmerz*) and are often utilized for treatment or even prevention of some forms of endometriosis (a painful condition resulting from abnormally located endometrial tissue).

Endometrial cancer. Several studies—both retrospective and prospective—have confirmed that the relative risk of endometrial cancer among pill users is less than half that of nonusers. It is unclear whether this effect continues after cessation of pill use.

Benign breast neoplasia (noncancerous tumors). Repeatedly, long-range studies have documented that pill takers are less likely to develop benign (noncancerous) tumors of the breast than women who do not use the pill. Some types of *existing* benign breast tumors can be aggravated by pill use, and therefore a breast mass is a relative contraindication.

Pelvic inflammatory disease. Many studies of pelvic inflammatory disease (PID) have shown a lower incidence of this potentially serious condition among users of oral contraceptives. The RCGP study found that the relative risk of PID among pill users was half that of nonusers (barrier methods of contraception may have a similar effect). A CDC study has confirmed that this protective effect has a significant public health impact: as many as 57,000 cases of PID may be averted each year in the United States by women using oral contraceptives.

There are at least two possible physiological explanations: the increased density of the cervical mucus in pill users may inhibit bacterial spread, and/or the pill's hormones may decrease the body's inflammatory response as other steroids are known to do.

Ectopic (tubal) pregnancy. Ectopic pregnancy is a potentially life-threatening condition. A large United States research study investigating the relationship of different contraceptive methods to the incidence of ectopic pregnancy found that *all* current users of a contraceptive method are less likely to have an ectopic pregnancy than are women who do not use contraception. The *lowest* incidence was among pill users, for whom the risk was only one-tenth that of women using no contraception. It is assumed that this protective effect is due to the pill's suppression of ovulation.

Arthritis. The large-scale RCGP study revealed the unexpected finding that the incidence of rheumatoid arthritis in pill users was half that in nonusers. This finding has now been confirmed in other studies. Although the mechanism for this effect is as yet unclear, protection against rheumatoid arthritis may be an attractive benefit of oral contraceptive use.

Iron-deficiency anemia. Because menstrual blood loss in oral contraceptive users is reduced by one-half on the average, pill use can reduce the incidence of iron deficiency anemia and therefore may be a good contraceptive choice for women with this type of anemia.

While the pill is being used for oral contraception, it may have additional beneficial effects for some patients. For example, acne, premenstrual tension, anxiety, or depression may be diminished by combined pills. In other women, however, all the above conditions might also be made somewhat worse by the use of oral contraceptives. Because of therapeutic hazards and extremely variable results, any use of oral contraceptives other than for contraceptive purposes should be undertaken only under the careful supervision and direction of a responsible physician.

SELECTION

Counseling Considerations

As described in Chapter 1, counseling the prospective contraceptive user is a complex, sensitive, and critically important process. Counseling is tied not only to client satisfaction, but to actual contraceptive effectiveness. The fact that, theoretically, oral contraceptives are nearly 100% effective in preventing pregnancy is sometimes compromised by high discontinuation rates—a high proportion of pill users stopping pill-taking after only a short period of time. The reasons for discontinuation are complex, but problems can be anticipated and prevented through careful counseling and education.

There are special considerations for the counselor-educator to be aware of when discussing the choice of oral contraception. Contraception is intimately connected with the client's sexuality. When taking oral contraceptives, the woman is reminded *daily* that she is assuming active responsibility for her reproductive planning. To the extent that the woman's partner can aid her in remembering to take the pill, this contraceptive method, like the barrier methods, offers an opportunity for partner involvement. In addition, unlike the intrauterine device (IUD), use of the pill requires a daily commitment to contraception. The efficacy of the method relies entirely on the woman's consistency in pill-taking.

Changes in menstrual patterns related to oral contraceptive use may have significant psychosocial implications. Some women may consider menstruation a cleansing of the body or may feel that their feminine identity is confirmed by regular menstruation. In such instances, scanty periods resulting from the use of oral contraceptives could make a woman feel less clean or less feminine than she felt prior to oral contraceptive use. In some cultures, women are expected to become pregnant immediately after marriage, alternating periods of lactation and pregnancy repeatedly, and menstruating rarely during their reproductive years as a result. Regular menstruation induced by oral contraceptive use can create anxiety for such a woman—an unexpected consequence of the pill's menstrual regularity.

Resistance to oral contraceptives may exist for surprisingly simple reasons. Some women may be wary of medicine in general. Others may be mistrustful of the pills themselves, being unused to the concept of health being obtained through oral tablets. One aspect of oral contraceptive use often regarded as a major advantage of the method is that it dissociates contraception from the sex act. However, some women may not understand how the pill can possibly prevent conception if it is not used in direct connection with intercourse. They may therefore take the pill improperly or not at all. As has been stressed, client comprehension of the pill's contraceptive mechanism, no matter how simply the concept is learned, can greatly help oral contraceptive acceptance and continuation.

The above discussion is not intended to imply that numerous psychosocial problems will complicate every woman's contraceptive decision. Indeed, many of these problems will never occur or cause serious rejection of oral contraceptives. Yet psychosocial aspects are important factors in client satisfaction, and the provider must be alert for potential difficulties.

Indications

Oral contraceptives are indicated for use by nonpregnant women who desire the most effective possible means of reversible contraception. The pill may be started after any menstrual period. It may be started immediately after abortion or in the immediate postpartum period for nonnursing mothers. If a mother wishes to nurse, use of oral contraceptives should be deferred for as long as she is breastfeeding and another form of contraception should be used. Certain pill formulations can be used in a special regimen when immediate postcoital contraception is required (see page 45).

The pill may be used for prevention of a first pregnancy or spacing of subsequent pregnancies, according to the woman's desires. The pill is particularly suitable for nulliparas (women who have not given birth), since the IUD is contraindicated in these women (see page 94). Sexually active adolescents who have established regular menstruation may take oral contraceptives.

Best current evidence indicates that the pill may be safely taken for many years, but for those women who have completed their family and definitely desire no further pregnancies, other long-term methods such as the IUD or sterilization should also be considered. There may be advantages, however, to long-term oral contraceptive use for some women. For example, some women may physically feel better when taking the pill than without it or may be concerned about obtaining the most effective protection from pregnancy that is possible without undergoing surgery. These conditions may justify long-term use of the pill, but because of increased potential complications, pill use by women over 40 years of age is not recommended (see page 62).

Contraindications

When oral contraceptives were first introduced, it was believed necessary to establish many rigid contraindications—physical conditions that should preclude the woman's use of the pill. Increasing experience with the safety and effectiveness of contraceptive pills has led to a marked reduction in absolute and relative contraindications to their use. *Absolute* contraindications are conditions that will cause a significant health risk to the client if the pill is taken. There

**Table 2-3.
Contraindications to Oral Contraceptives.**

Absolute	Relative
Thrombophlebitis	Significant hypertension
Thromboembolism	Severe migraine
Stroke	Age over 35 years
Coronary artery disease	Tobacco smoking
Serious liver disease	Cervical dysplasia
Pregnancy	Diabetes
Cancer of breasts or	Gallbladder disease
reproductive system	

is some disagreement among family planning physicians, but in general the most widely accepted absolute contraindications to oral contraceptive use are the following (see also Table 2-3):

Thrombophlebitis (blood clot in an inflamed vein) or thrombo-embolism (moving blood clot) or a history of these conditions. Thrombophlebitis is characterized by persistent pelvic or leg pain, with accompanying inflammation and swelling of the skin over a deep vein. This contraindication does not include uncomplicated varicose veins.

Thromboembolism is characterized by sudden severe chest pain associated with the coughing up of blood, acute shortness of breath, irregular heartbeat, and respiratory insufficiency followed by persistent pleuritic pain (painful breathing).

Cerebrovascular accident (stroke) or a history of this condition. A cerebrovascular accident (CVA) is caused by either a blood clot or a rupture in a brain blood vessel. It is characterized by the symptoms of stroke—severe headache, loss of consciousness, and disruptions of motor and sensory function.

Coronary artery disease or a history of this condition. Because of the increased risk of myocardial infarction (heart attack) associated with pill use (see page 61), a history of coronary artery disease is a contraindication to pill use. The clinician will rarely find such a history in young women, however.

Serious diseases of the liver. Such diseases include cirrohsis, chronic liver insufficiency, extensive parasitic infestations involving the liver, hepatic adenoma, and a history of cholestatic jaundice during pregnancy. The presence of a significantly enlarged liver or ascites (fluid collection in the abdominal cavity) or the presence of jaundice are conditions that may be visible on examination and are contraindications to pill use. In the presence of these conditions, the hormones in the oral contraceptives will be metabolized more slowly, possibly making the pill's side-effects more pronounced. Primary or secondary liver tumors are also contraindications to pill use.

Known or suspected malignancy of the breasts or reproductive system. Only estrogen-dependent malignancies are absolute contraindications to pill use. Despite the efforts of many clinical studies, no association (either positive or negative) has been found between breast cancer and oral contraceptive use. Nevertheless, pre-existing breast cancer is a serious condition and can become worse if the patient takes the pill. Endometrial cancer is the only other common cancer type that is a contraindication to pill use. Paradoxically, pill use is apparently *protective* against the *development* of endometrial carcinoma as well as ovarian cancer (see page 28). Adenocarcinoma (cancer) of the cervix is a rare condition more typical of postmenopausal women and thus will probably not be seen by the family planning worker. This condition would also be an absolute contraindication to pill use if found.

Known or suspected pregnancy. If the woman is known or suspected to be pregnant, she should discontinue oral contraceptive use immediately because of possible effects of the pill on the fetus (see page 67).

There are also *relative* contraindications to oral contraceptive use that must be carefully considered (by a physician, if possible), including:

Significant hypertension. There is no absolute level of elevated blood pressure that contraindicates oral contraceptive use. This must be weighed in the context of what is considered locally significant hypertension, accounting for the effects of age and geography on this condition. It is generally recommended that a blood pressure over 140/90 mm Hg be considered high, meriting special monitoring and care in follow-up of the patient.

Oral contraceptives may also be associated with the *development* of hypertension in some women, and hypertension is known to be a predisposing factor to cardiovascular disease. The pill can reveal this potential health hazard for a patient who is predisposed to hypertension. Women with other predisposing factors, such as to-bacco smoking, obesity, and diabetes, might consider another effec-tive method of contraception, if available. It should be kept in mind that pregnancy can also induce a rise in blood pressure. Research has shown that it is not possible to predict which women will de-velop hypertension while on the pill. Fortunately, such pill-revealed hypertension usually disappears after oral contraceptive use is stopped.

Severe and frequent migraine headache. *Migraine* is defined as a strong, throbbing headache usually preceded by visual distur-bance and accompanied by nausea. It is often relieved by sleep. This type of headache is caused by a vessel spasm and is definitely a contraindication to oral contraceptive use. Headache can also be psychosomatic—caused by psychological or emotional stress in the patient—in which case pills can be continued unless these symp-toms are severe and become worse during pill use. Careful judgment of the patient's headache is necessary in order to determine whether oral contraceptives can be safely continued. Proper follow-up is critical (see page 49).

Age and tobacco smoking. Circulatory system diseases have been shown convincingly to be more likely to occur in women who are older (generally over 35 years of age) or who smoke tobacco. Both factors—age and smoking—together produce a synergistic (greater than additive) increased risk. Women over 30, and espe-cially over 35, should be advised of these risks, and the available contraceptive alternatives should be carefully reviewed. Smoking, of course, is a serious health hazard to all humans and is incompatible with safe use of oral contraceptives.

Cervical dysplasia. A recent study has implied that pill use may promote the progression of preexisting cervical dysplasia (non-malignant abnormal cells) to carcinoma in situ (a precancerous con-dition). This study did *not* find the pill *causing* dysplasia. Further research is necessary to confirm or refute this association, but cervi-cal dysplasia may be considered by some to be a relative contraindi-cation to oral contraceptive use.

Diabetes mellitus. Diabetes is a relative contraindication to pill use only to the degree that this condition serves as a predispos-ing risk factor to circulatory system disease. The provider and the patient should weigh the benefits and risks carefully and realistically in this situation. For a younger nonsmoking woman in whom diabetes is the only extra risk factor, oral contraceptives may still be an acceptable contraceptive choice. For an older obese smoker, having diabetes as well would probably rule out any use of the pill. The clinician must remember that pregnancy in diabetes is a high-risk condition. Consequently, excluding those women with other risk factors, pill-taking may be the preferred risk in diabetics who need an effective means of preventing pregnancy.

Diabetes itself is not made worse by oral contraceptive use, although there is a reduction of glucose tolerance among pill-takers. Prediabetic patients may therefore develop overt symptoms of diabetes earlier on oral contraceptives than if they had not taken them. Prediabetics may be suspected by being overweight, by a history of large babies (over 4000 g birth weight) or by a family history of diabetes. Overt diabetics may require more insulin while on oral contraceptives, and thus pill use in diabetics requires careful physician supervision.

Gallbladder disease. It is unclear whether pill-taking is associated with gallbladder disease, but use of oral contraceptives may uncover this condition in susceptible women (see page 65). A history of gallbladder disease should thus be considered a relative contraindication to pill use.

Misunderstandings and Cautions

The conditions discussed in the preceding paragraphs encompass the major absolute and relative contraindications to oral contraceptive use. It is important to clarify several other misunderstandings:

Chronic mild hypertension. There is no contraindication to pill-taking among chronic *mild* hypertensives, if it is demonstrated by repeated blood pressure tests that the hypertension *remains* mild on the pill. Indeed, this mild condition may occasionally show improvement during oral contraceptive use, either spontaneously or over time.

Cancer. There is no evidence of the pill *causing* cancer. In fact, oral contraceptive use apparently *protects* against the development of endometrial and ovarian cancer. Any cancer that is not estrogen-dependent will *not* be worsened by oral contraceptive use, including leukemia and most cases of cancer of the lung, thyroid, stomach, colon, skin, connective tissue, bone, or brain. Any known malignancy that is found should, of course, be treated by a physician.

Thyroid disorders. These conditions, including hypo- or hyperthyroidism, thyroiditis, or smooth or nodular goiter, are not a contraindication to oral contraceptive use. Nevertheless, they are all conditions that warrant appropriate diagnosis and therapy.

Sexually transmitted diseases. Sexually transmitted diseases such as gonorrhea or syphilis are not a contraindication to oral contraceptive use. These diseases are very serious, however, and demand immediate attention.

Other conditions have at one time or another been considered possible contraindications to oral contraceptives, and local decisions should be made about their applicability. These conditions include severe varicose veins, epilepsy, and a menstrual history suggestive of potential infertility problems—such as delay in the adolescent onset of menstruation (menarche) or irregular menstruation.

It should be reiterated that in many situations when the pill is the only reasonable effective means of available contraception, it may be desirable for women with significant medical problems to take oral contraceptives rather than risk the greater health hazards from pregnancy. Diseases that may be worsened by pregnancy include hypertension, liver and kidney disease, heart disease, and epilepsy. The risk of circulatory problems, including thrombophlebitis, embolism, and CVA, may also be worsened by pregnancy more severely than by oral contraceptive use. Thus pill use may be preferable to the unwanted pregnancy that might occur without it. This is especially true in those areas where maternal mortality is high.

Pill Selection

History. Any woman who is considering oral contraceptives should have a medical history recorded to check for potential problems with the pill. This history is very important and is more significant than physical examination in determining contraindications to pill-taking. The medical history can be easily taken through a few short questions by a trained health worker and should focus on areas of absolute and relative contraindications. If absolute contraindications such as a history of thromboembolism are present, the woman should not use oral contraceptives. If relative contrain-

Table 2-4. Sample Questions for History-Taking.
Have you ever had:
• Severe headaches?
• Yellow skin or eyes?
• Palpable breast mass?
• Discharge from the nipple?
• Severe chest pains?
• Unusual shortness of breath or fatigue after exertion?
• Prolonged or frequent menstruation?
• Bleeding after sexual intercourse?
• Swelling or severe pain in legs?

dications are present, the patient should be seen by a physician before oral contraceptives are prescribed. Simple history questionnaires have been used successfully in a large number of family planning programs (Table 2-4). When a family planning clinic prepares its own questionnaire and guidelines to the interview process, the language should be carefully written so as to be the most understandable to both the health worker and the client.

It is impossible to predict with certainty which pill users will experience side-effects. A few simple questions about the woman's experience during menstruation and pregnancy, plus observation of body build, can simplify the selection of the proper contraceptive pill. For example, a woman's experiences on the pill are likely to be similar to her experiences during pregnancy, except in a lesser degree. If she had nausea and vomiting during a previous pregnancy, she can be expected to have a milder version of these problems for a few months after starting pill use. Her body needs time to adapt to the new levels of hormones. Similarly, a woman with a history of heavy menstruation or dysmenorrhea may experience more problems with irregular bleeding during the first several months of adjustment to pill use than do those women with a history of normal flow.

If a woman is advised and reassured about the possibility of side-effects, her acceptance and continuation of oral contraceptive use may be easier, or she may prefer from the outset to choose another contraceptive method. The provider should also be aware that occasionally the very discussion of some side-effects with the woman before she starts oral contraceptives may contribute to the occurrence and reporting of these effects or may cause unnecessary anxiety. This is one of the delicate factors the provider must balance when dealing individually with each client.

Table 2-5.
Physical Examination of Prospective Pill Users.

- General observation; establish baseline characteristics
- Check blood pressure
- Palpate breasts and liver edge
- *Optional:* routine pelvic examination; Pap smear

Examination. If possible, a general physical examination is desirable before dispensing oral contraceptives (Table 2-5). This examination should consist of general observation of the general organic condition, blood pressure test, and palpation of the breasts (Figure 2-4) and liver edge (Figure 2-5). With the exception of elevated blood pressure and palpable breast nodules, most conditions where cautious oral contraceptive use is advisable are disclosed by history and not by physical examination. The physical examination does establish the woman's baseline physical characteristics for future reference in the management of any potential problems.

Pelvic examination is not mandatory for oral contraceptive use. Having the patient in the health clinic for provision of family planning services may be an excellent opportunity for a routine pelvic examination, however. This examination can include a check for cervicitis, vaginitis, abnormalities of the pelvic organs, and a cervical cytology test for uterine cancer screening (Papanicolaou or "Pap" smear) where medical personnel and facilities warrant it.

As a practical matter, routine pelvic examinations will not appreciably increase the chances of diagnosing conditions that contraindicate oral contraceptive use and will not reduce complications from use of the pill. Insistence on a pelvic examination may be counterproductive in those cultures where women have an aversion to such examinations or where the health care system does not have the resources to conduct them.

Pill Formulas

The two major types of oral contraceptive preparations currently used most frequently worldwide provide excellent contraceptive effectiveness for most women without undue discomfort from side-effects. The two preparations that we focus on fall at each end of the currently acceptable range of hormonal dosages. The first consists of 1 mg of the progestin norethindrone and 50 µg of the estrogen mestranol (Norinyl or Noriday 1/50, Syntex and Ortho-

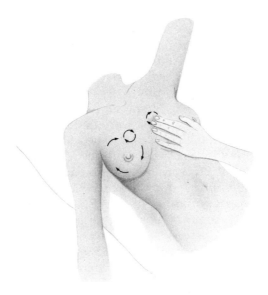

Figure 2-4. *To palpate the breast to check for an abnormal mass, the examiner's hand should move in a small circular motion clockwise around the breast.*

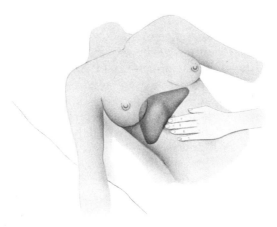

Figure 2-5. *Palpation of the liver edge can help detect contraindications to pill use.*

Novum 1/50, Ortho). This oral contraceptive preparation has been widely distributed for many years. The second preparation is representative of the pills more recently marketed to achieve safe and effective contraceptive protection with the minimum hormonal dose. This pill contains 0.5 mg of norethindrone with 35 µg of the estrogen ethinyl estradiol (Brevicon or Norminest, Syntex and Modicon, Ortho). In this book, the first pill is referred to as the "1/50" pill and the second, as the "low-dose" pill (see Table 2-1). Selecting which preparation to use is discussed in detail in this section.

When oral contraceptives were first introduced in 1960, it was thought that hormone levels had to be as high as those in pregnancy in order to provide maximum contraceptive effectiveness. However, the high dose of estrogen in early preparations led to a number of side-effects, the most serious of which was thromboembolism. Since 1969 the Royal Committee on the Safety of Drugs in the United Kingdom has recommended that patients be started on pills containing 50 µg of estrogen or less to minimize the possibility of thromboembolism. In 1970, the U.S. Food and Drug Administration (FDA) made a similar statement, recommending use of "the lowest effective dose of estrogen that is otherwise acceptable." Modern lower-dose preparations have resulted in blood levels of hormones that are about the same as those in the latter part of the normal menstrual cycle. As a result, side-effects of all types have been reduced while contraceptive effectiveness has been maintained.

The lesser amounts of estrogen and progestin in the low-dose pills cause a lower incidence of some side-effects in pill users and a higher incidence of others. Whereas circulatory effects may be reduced, breakthrough bleeding and other menstrual irregularities may be increased. The risk of unwanted conceptions occurring because of interrupted pill-taking is also slightly higher with low-dose pills. A recent international meeting of family planning researchers and administrators concluded that in light of the bleeding problems and pregnancy risks, low-dose pills were ideal for clinic-based pill programs but were less suitable for community-based or commercial nonclinical distribution common in many developing countries. Where the proper clinical referral system is available, however, the use of both 1/50 and low-dose pills gives a family planning service useful flexibility.

Most women can be effectively protected from pregnancy with a minimum amount of contraceptive hormones, and both the 1/50 and the low-dose pills are excellent preparations for almost all women who do not have contraindications. In helping the woman select a

Table 2-6. Guidelines for Initial Choice: Low-Dose Versus 1/50 Pills.	
Low-Dose	**1/50**
Slender to moderate build	Moderate to heavy build
Regular menstrual cycles	Menstrual irregularity
Reliable pill-taking	Less reliable pill-taking
Clear complexion	Acne

pill preparation, the provider should judge the woman's physical and behavioral characteristics, medical history, and the relative availability of the pill formulations (see Table 2-6). If the woman is of slender to moderate build, generally healthy with regular menstrual cycles, and can be relied on to take the pill every day, the low-dose pill is an excellent choice. If the woman is more obese, has acne, or has a history of menstrual irregularity, she many benefit from the higher estrogen dose in the 1/50 pill. Also, any provider who believes that the woman will be less dependable in taking the pill should recommend the 1/50 pill, since the risk of conception if pill-taking is interrupted is higher with the low-dose pills. As can be seen from this discussion, the provider and client should have at least two pill formulations available from which to choose.

There are numerous other oral contraceptive preparations currently being used around the world containing different synthetic hormones in different doses and combinations. In combined pills, the estrogen component in most oral contraceptives is either mestranol or ethinyl estradiol, and both are very similar in their effects.

The progestins used vary greatly (Table 2-7). Norethindrone is a moderately progestational substance that has no compounding estrogenic effects. Norgestrel, which has nonestrogenic and strong progestational properties, making the pills containing it somewhat different in hormonal influence from other pills. Norgestrel is found in pills of standard and low-dose formulations. Another common oral contraceptive progestin is norethindrone acetate used in varying doses, usually with ethinyl estradiol. Norethindrone acetate is an active progestin with androgenic and antiestrogenic effects. Ethynodiol diacetate, another common progestin, exerts an estrogenic influence and thus compounds the effect of the estrogen in the pill. Lynestrenol is still another progestin used in some oral contraceptives, combined with ethinyl estradiol.

Table 2-7.
Oral Contraceptive Formulas by Dosages and Brand Names.

Progestin (mg)	Estrogen (μg)	Brand Name
Ethynodiol diacetate 1.0	Mestranol 100	Ovulen
Norethindrone 1.0	Mestranol 50	Norinyl 1/50, Noriday, Ortho-Novum 1/50
Norethindrone 0.4	Ethinyl estradiol 35	Ovcon 35
Norethindrone 0.5	Ethinyl estradiol 35	Brevicon, Modicon, Norminest
Norethindrone 1.0	Ethinyl estradiol 35	Norinyl 1/35, Ortho-Novum 1/35
Norethindrone 1.0	Ethinyl estradiol 50	Ovcon 50
Norgestrel 0.15	Ethinyl estradiol 30	Microgynon, Ovranette
Norgestral 0.25	Ethinyl estradiol 30	Eugynon 30, Ovran 30
Norgestrel 0.30	Ethinyl estradiol 30	Lo-ovral
Norgestrel 0.25	Ethinyl estradiol 50	Eugynon 50, Ovran 50
Norgestrel 0.50	Ethinyl estradiol 50	Ovral
Norethindrone acetate 1.0	Ethinyl estradiol 20	Loestrin 1/20, Zorane 1/20
Norethindrone acetate 1.5	Ethinyl estradiol 30	Loestrin 1.5/30, Zorane 1.5/30
Norethindrone acetate 1.0	Ethinyl estradiol 50	Norlestrin 1/50, Zorane 1/50, Minovlar
Norethindrone acetate 3.0	Ethinyl estradiol 50	Gynovlar 1/50,
Norethindrone acetate 4.0	Ethinyl estradiol 50	Anovlar
Ethynodiol diacetate 2.0	Ethinyl estradiol 30	Conova 30
Ethynodiol diacetate 1.0	Ethinyl estradiol 35	Demulen 1/35
Ethynodiol diacetate 1.0	Ethinyl estradiol 50	Demulen 1/50
Lynestrenol 1.0	Ethinyl estradiol 50	Ovostat
Lynestrenal 2.5	Ethinyl estradiol 50	Minilyn

Brand Name	Estrogen (μg)	Progestin (mg)	
Anovlar	EE 50	NA	4.0
Brevicon	EE 35	N	0.5
Conova 30	EE 30	ED	2.0
Demulen 1/35, 1/50	EE 35,50	ED	1.0
Eugynon 30, 50	EE 30,50	Norg	0.25
Gynovlar	EE 50	NA	3.0
Loestrin 1.5/30, 1/20	EE 30,20	NA	1.5, 1.0
Lo-ovral	EE 30	Norg	0.30
Microgynon	EE 30	Norg	0.15
Minilyn	EE 50	Lyn	2.5
Minovlar	EE 50	NA	1.0
Modicon	EE 35	N	0.5
Norinyl 1/35, 1/50	M 35,50	N	1.0
Norlestrin 1/50	EE 50	NA	1.0
Ortho-Novum 1/35, 1/50	M 35,50	N	1.0
Ovcon 35, 50	EE 35,50	N	0.4,1.0
Ovostat	EE 50	Lyn	1.0
Ovral	EE 50	Norg	0.5
Ovran 30, 50	EE 30,50	Norg.	0.25
Ovranette	EE 30	Norg	0.15
Ovulen	M 100	ED	1.0
Zorane 1/20, 1.5/30, 1/50	EE 20,30,50	NA	1.0,1.5,1.0

EE = ethinyl estradiol, M = mestranol, NA = norethindrone acetate, N = norethindrone, ED = ethnodiol diacete, Norg = norgestrel, Lyn = lynstrenol.

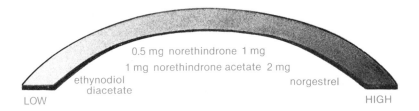

Figure 2-6. *Spectrum of progestational potency.*

An important concept for the clinician to understand is relative progestational *potency.* Potency varies according to the characteristics described above, and also by dosage. Progestational potency is receiving increasing attention as a factor in possible circulatory disease complications from pill use (see page 59). To simplify the discussion, commonly used progestins can be divided into high- and low-potency categories. The following can be considered to be high-potency progestin formulations: norgestrel 0.5 and 0.25 mg, norethindrone 1 mg, and norethindrone acetate 2 mg. Formulations with low progestational potency are norethindrone 0.5 mg, norethindrone acetate 1 mg, and ethynodiol diacetate 1 and 2 mg (Figure 2-6).

This description of oral contraceptive preparations is presented without a detailed discussion of their subtle pharmacological distinctions or clinical uses. Nevertheless, this information should aid any clinician who is providing oral contraceptives other than the two formulations we have chosen for discussion in this chapter.

Pill-Taking

Each woman should be carefully instructed about taking oral contraceptives before beginning her pill regimen. This counseling will help prevent any misunderstanding that may be personally troublesome for the client and will enable her to use the pill confidently and correctly.

Some pills are provided in 28-day cycle cards (Figure 2-7), which have been found to be less confusing than other regimens for women just starting the pill. The pills are usually arranged in four rows of seven pills each—one row for each week of use. The woman should start taking her pills on the fifth day after the start of her menstrual period. She should take one pill every day in the package sequence and should always take it around the same time of day, such as when first waking up in the morning or before going to bed. After the first 21 pills are taken, the woman should continue without

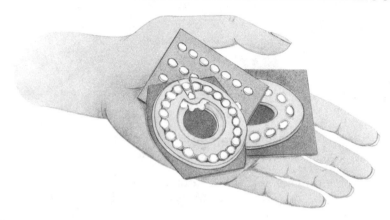

Figure 2-7. *Oral contraceptives come in different styles of pill cards, in 21-day or 28-day regimens.*

interruption taking the next 7 pills, which are usually of a different color and contain 75 mg of iron (but no hormones). This iron (ferrous fumarate) dose is considerably below levels of supplementary iron necessary for treatment of anemia but is given rather than a placebo to help counteract chronic iron deficiency found in many women.

When pills are supplied in 21-day cards, the woman begins pill-taking in the same manner. But after 21 pills are taken consecutively, she must wait 7 consecutive days before beginning a new cycle card. This regimen obviously requires more care in remembering proper pill-taking and more care in client instruction.

The onset of menstruation should occur during the week the woman is off the hormonal regimen. If she is using the 28-day cycle, the woman should go on to the pills from the next cycle card, without interruption. This is usually coincident with the cessation of menstruation, but even if the flow has not stopped, the new package should be begun anyway. Thus with the 28-day regimen, a pill is taken every single day of the year. If she is using the 21-day cycle, the woman begins taking pills from the new cycle card 7 days after taking the last pill, whether or not she has menstruated.

Oral contraceptives are only as effective as the ability of the woman to remember to take them; forgetfulness may lead to pregnancy. There is no precise time of each day when pills should be taken, but it is desirable to instruct the woman to take her pills daily at roughly the same time. This results in more stable hormone levels in the body and, furthermore, will make pill-taking easier to remember. If pill-taking is made part of an already existing habit, such as the evening meal or preparing for bed, consistency will be enhanced. Some have suggested that the partner be included in the responsibility of remembering to take the daily pill while the habit is first being learned. Innovative methods for remembering can be developed for differing cultural situations.

Theoretically, the woman will not get pregnant during her first cycle of pills if she starts pill-taking on day 5 of menstruation. Because of possible subjective problems such as forgetfulness in adjusting to pill-taking, some practitioners suggest the use of another contraceptive method such as condoms or foam through the first cycle of pill use. On the other hand, temporary use of two contraceptive methods can be confusing, add unnecessary expense, and end up irritating the client, resulting in discontinuation of pill use altogether. Once again, this is a situation requiring independent judgment by the woman and her provider.

Postpartum and postabortion. In the postpartum period, the woman can begin her pills immediately if she is not nursing her infant. If she is nursing, the mother should be advised to wait until she finishes breastfeeding. In some cases pill use may reduce milk production or the hormones may be secreted in the mother's milk. The breast milk in pill users may be of higher quality, however, according to a recent Bangladesh study. If there is an interval between birth of the newborn and the beginning of pill use, another means of contraception should be employed to avoid any possibility of accidental pregnancy while awaiting the first postpartum menstruation.

Women who have had a recent abortion or stillbirth should start pill use *immediately* without waiting for a menstrual period. They will have their menstrual periods regularly once pill use is begun. Immediate postabortal use is important because ovulation begins again so quickly. According to one study, ovulation returns in three-fourths of postabortal women within 6 weeks.

Postcoital. A family planning provider will often first see a woman when she has just had unprotected intercourse, usually at midcycle, and she does not want to become pregnant. Until recently, the provider has only been able to advise the woman to "wait and see" or to prescribe high doses of estrogen in order to intercept implantation, neither of which is satisfactory. The provider now has two choices that are much safer, very effective, and that can start the woman on long-term pregnancy prevention. One method is the postcoital insertion of an IUD (see page 97), and the other is a special regimen of a specific oral contraceptive formulation.

The recommended regimen for prevention of pregnancy in the immediate postcoital period (within 72 hours) is *two* pills containing the progestin norgestrel and an estrogen (Ovral, Eugynon), taken simultaneously, followed by another two pills 12 hours later. The failure rate for this regimen has been found to be less than 1%, and the major side-effect—nausea and vomiting—although frequent (60%), is less severe than with high-estrogen regimens. Symptoms generally pass within 72 hours; routine administration of antiemetics is probably not necessary. It is possible that other pill formulations could be used in a similar manner, but their safety and effectiveness have not yet been documented.

There is the theoretical risk that in cases of failure (less than 1%), the resulting fetus may have congenital malformations because of exposure to the concentrated hormonal dose. This risk is probably lower than that with the high-estrogen regimen. Nevertheless, administration of the pill for postcoital contraception may not be appropriate for women who, in case of method failure, would not consider termination of the resulting unwanted pregnancy.

During the initial visit for postcoital contraception, the provider should emphasize the importance of regular use of effective contraception, and the full range of available methods should be explained. This is an excellent opportunity to start the client in family planning.

Missing pills. Every woman needs to be counseled before beginning pill-taking so that all questions and potential problems are dealt with satisfactorily. Side-effects of the pill must be discussed thoroughly, yet without inducing unnecessary anxiety. And each woman must be carefully instructed about what to do if she forgets to take her pills.

The following instructions are for women taking the 1/50 pill (see also Table 2-8). If one pill is not taken at the usual time, the woman should take that pill as soon as she remembers and then take the next pill as usual. The same applies if she misses two pills. Slight breakthrough bleeding or nausea may be noted because of disturbance of the dose pattern. If the woman misses three pills, the chance of ovulation occurring is increased, and another form of contraception should be used immediately. No more pills should be taken, and the client should await the onset of menstrual-like bleeding that is expected. The woman recommences pill-taking with a new cycle card beginning 7 days after the last pill was taken.

Table 2-8. Missed Pills: Client Instructions.

1/50 pill:
Missed 1—take when you remember and continue pill-taking
Missed 2—as above
Missed 3—STOP pill-taking; use another contraceptive method;
    resume pill-taking in 7 days
 	
Low-dose or 1/35 pill:
Missed 1—take when you remember and continue pill-taking
Missed 2—STOP pill-taking; use another contraceptive method;
    resume pill-taking in 7 days

If the woman is taking the low-dose pills, however, the risk of pregnancy as a result of interrupting regular pill-taking is greater than with the 1/50 pills. If the woman misses one low-dose pill, she should take that pill as soon as she remembers and take the next pill as usual. But if she misses two pills, she should immediately begin using another form of contraception and recommence pill-taking with a new cycle card as described above. This protocol also applies to women using the 1/35 formulations.

A study by Guillebaud in England has found that, contrary to common expectations, the greatest risk of pregnancy when pill-taking is interrupted occurs when the pill is missed around the *beginning* or *end* of the cycle, *not* in midcycle. His research shows that a high level of the natural hormone estradiol occurs in some women by the end of the 7 pill-free days (or 7 placebo days if using a 28-day regimen). This suggests a "preovulatory" state. If a pill or two are missed around this time, it adds to the number of days the body is without external hormonal influence. This increases the risk of an LH surge, which could induce ovulation. In midcycle, a missed pill entails only a 1- or 2-day interruption, at a time when estradiol levels are quite low. This does not give the body enough time to begin normal hormonal impulses to induce ovulation.

These findings make it important for the oral contraceptive user to realize that conscientious pill-taking is even more important around the *pill-free* (or placebo) week than at other times—the opposite of what she might have assumed (Figure 2-8). This research also might suggest a more cautious approach if a woman misses two 1/50 pills around the week of menstruation: start extra contraceptive protection immediately while awaiting the 7 days to pass before beginning a new pill cycle.

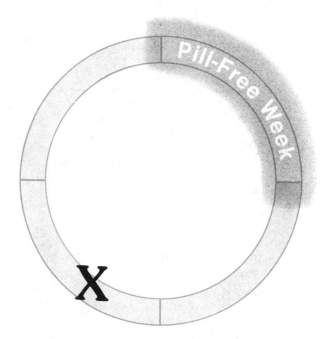

Figure 2-8. *The period of highest risk of pregnancy from interrupted pill-taking is just before and just after the pill-free week, not at midcycle as is usually assumed.*

It is important to emphasize that if the woman has been taking her pills correctly and misses a menstrual period, there is little need for concern and pill use can be continued normally. The woman is most likely adjusting to lower hormone levels in her body. If she misses two periods while correctly taking the pill, the woman should contact her clinician for an examination. The practitioner must recognize and carefully explain to the client that menstrual bleeding during the pill may be very short and scanty. One or two days of light spotting at the time of expected menstruation can be validly interpreted as menstruation and not amenorrhea. However, if the woman has *not* been taking her pills correctly and has missed a menstrual period, the possibility of pregnancy is greater and a pregnancy test should be performed.

FOLLOW-UP

Follow-up of women taking oral contraceptives is extremely important. There can be a high discontinuation rate if minor problems are not dealt with and if appropriate reassurance is not provided.

The risk of developing serious complications can also be reduced by prompt recognition of potential symptoms. Procedures for follow-up will vary according to locality, but in general they are best conducted when patients are seen for resupply of pills.

Follow-Up Visits

The initial return visit should usually be at 3 months, when blood pressure should be taken and pelvic and breast examination performed if previous abnormalities were noted. The pill user should be questioned regarding symptoms suggestive of phlebitis or other vascular problems while on the pill. Minor problems of any sort should be promptly resolved and the client given reassurance when necessary.

The early follow-up visit is needed to check on proper pill-taking as well as possible side-effects. It is important to determine whether the woman is taking her pills properly. Simple mistakes are surprisingly common and may be the cause of completely unnecessary pill discontinuation. Even inconsistent pill-taking can eliminate the pill's high degree of effectiveness and result in unwanted pregnancy.

After the initial follow-up visit, assuming no abnormalities have been detected, the woman need not be seen until the end of the first year of pill use, unless clinic visits are necessary for resupply or interim problems arise. The annual examination should include an interim history, physical examination including blood pressure, breast and liver edge palpation (Figures 2-4 and 2-5), and pelvic examination with Pap smear, provided these are appropriate for the clinical setting.

Events that may occur after beginning oral contraceptive use can be categorized as either *side-effects*—normally anticipated events associated with pill use without serious danger to the woman's health—or *complications*—abnormal events that are not generally anticipated and that may endanger the woman's health.

Side-Effects and Management

Since oral contraceptives may provide more or less estrogen and progestin than the woman's body has been accustomed to, some women may have side-effects from the pill with varying degrees of intensity. For the first several cycles of pill-taking, side-effects may be particularly troublesome, including nausea and occasionally vomiting and breakthrough bleeding or spotting during the cycle. These reactions result from changes in the woman's hormonal environ-

Table 2-9. Side-Effects of Oral Contraceptives.	
Definitely Attributable	**Possibly Attributable**
Breakthrough bleeding	Headache
Scant menstruation	Depression
Urinary tract infection	Mastalgia
Vaginal discharge and irritation	Weight change
Chloasma	Libido change

ment. One symptom or another usually occurs in up to 25% of pill users during the first cycle but diminishes rapidly so that only about 5% of the women will experience any side-effects after three cycles of pill use. Each pill user must be reassured that these symptoms are not unusual or serious. Otherwise she may stop taking the pills almost immediately after beginning them, without allowing sufficient time for side-effects to disappear.

Although side-effects do deserve recognition from the clinician, some women may feel that numerous physical symptoms occurring during pill use are caused by the pill, when in fact they may not be. Thus side-effects may be *definitely attributable* or *possibly attributable* to the pill (Table 2-9). Frequently noted side-effects *definitely attributable* to oral contraceptive use are:

Continuing breakthrough bleeding. Mild intermenstrual spotting during the first several cycles of pill-taking is common and not alarming. Heavier breakthrough bleeding can be a more difficult problem that requires careful management. Breakthrough bleeding is caused by relative estrogen deficiency and can usually be controlled on the days it occurs by having the women take two contraceptive pills per day for several days. The woman should take the extra pills from a separate cycle card obtained from the provider. This method is called *doubling-up* and simply provides additional estrogen to curtail unwanted intermenstrual bleeding.

If the woman has started on a low-dose pill and despite doubling-up has persistent problems with breakthrough bleeding after several cycles, her regimen should be changed to a preparation with more estrogen (a 1/50 pill).

If there is significant breakthrough bleeding in a woman initially started on a higher estrogen dose (a 1/50 pill), doubling-up can again be used. If the bleeding is still unresponsive when the dose is doubled, it may be necessary to discontinue the pills and use another method of contraception. Continued maintenance of a patient on double doses of a 1/50 pill is unacceptable and not recommended.

Scant menstruation. This is a common problem related to the use of contraceptive pills. Menstruation may be significantly diminished or even absent (amenorrhea) when a woman is taking oral contraceptives. If a woman has been taking her pills regularly and properly, scant menstruation usually does not mean that an unwanted pregnancy has occurred. Even just 1 or 2 days of light spotting during the week that menstruation is expected can be validly interpreted as a menstrual equivalent, and the patient should be given appropriate reassurance. If two menstrual periods are missed completely, the woman should be examined. If continuing scant menstruation is disturbing for the patient, she may need additional estrogen and can have her condition improved by a switch from a low-dose to a 1/50 pill or to a pill containing norgestrel.

Urinary tract infection. The large prospective study by the Royal College of General Practitioners (RCGP) found an increased incidence of urinary tract infection (UTI) among oral contraceptive users than in nonusers. Cystitis, for instance, was reported 20% more often in pill users than in nonusers in that study (56 per 1000 woman-years versus 46 per 1000 in controls). The Walnut Creek study, which has followed over 16,000 Californian pill users since the early 1970s, also found a significant increase in the risk of UTI among pill users of all ages. Both studies believe these findings are due to increased sexual activity during oral contraceptive use, rather than from an actual effect of the pill itself. Women with urinary tract infection while on the pill can continue taking oral contraceptives but should receive appropriate treatment.

Vaginal discharge and irritation. Some women may have increased vaginal discharge while taking oral contraceptives. There is disagreement whether this is a direct effect of the pills or a secondary effect from the woman's possibly increased sexual activity. The woman should be examined if there is a complaint of discharge, and should receive appropriate treatment if vaginitis is evident. If she is having continuing problems with moniliasis (yeast infection) while on the low-dose pill, a change to a higher-estrogen preparation (1/50 pill) may also be helpful.

Chloasma. Chloasma is increased facial skin pigmentation, similar to the so-called mask of pregnancy. This condition may be diminished by having the patient keep out of the sun or use vanishing creams, but may take a very long time to disappear. Since chloasma has been found to be related to estrogen levels, its incidence is rare with modern preparations.

Some symptoms described by women taking oral contraceptives cannot be definitely attributed to the pill. These include symptoms such as headache, depression, breast pain (mastalgia), weight changes and bloating, and loss of sex drive (libido). These are common concerns among pill-takers, but have no definite statistical association with pill use. The *possibly attributable* side-effects include:

Headache. Headache is a common complaint in any human being and can be due to a myriad of factors. The importance of caution when managing migraine headache in pill users has been discussed previously. Seeking the cause of a particular patient's headache requires some sophistication in diagnosis. Headaches observed in pill users will generally be caused either by migraine, hypertension, or anxiety. The goal in sorting through the symptoms is to determine whether the headache is vascular (migraine), in which case pill use should be stopped.

Symptoms at the onset of the headache and their response to analgesics can be helpful in determining the cause of headache. It is important to know whether the patient's headache started or be-

---

Table 2-10.
Questions for Differential Diagnosis
of Headache in Pill Users.

- Worse in past 48 hours?
- Usually last one hour or longer?
- Started or become worse since starting pill?
- Accompanied by dizziness, nausea or vomiting?
- Accompanied by spots in front of the eyes, watery eyes, blurred vision, or loss of vision?
- History of hypertension?
- Usually occur on one side of the head?
- Throbbing?
- Continue after taking painkiller?
- Personal or family history of migraine headache?

Adapted from Contraceptive Technology Update, June 1980.

came worse since beginning pill use. Severity is another important parameter, although a subjective one. One test for severity is to ask if the patient feels the headaches are "interfering with her life." The Emory University Family Planning Program has developed a useful questionnaire to aid in the differential diagnosis of headaches (Table 2-10). The patient completes the questions on her own before seeing the clinician; this technique elicits a very complete set of relevant symptomatic information.

After this careful evaluation, if migraine is suspected or if the headaches are severe and continuing, oral contraceptives should be discontinued and the patient carefully evaluated.

Depression. Depression is also a very common human experience, and is difficult to study in relation to pill use. Recent research results have reached conflicting conclusions about pill use and depression. Some increased incidence or intensity of depression in women on the pill may be due to a pill-induced deficiency of pyridoxine (vitamin B_6). This deficiency can disturb some metabolic processes and upset normal neurological function, perhaps causing depressive symptoms. The frequency of a clinically significant pyridoxine deficiency due to pill use is probably very low.

Mastalgia. Breast tenderness or pain occurs in many women during the normal menstrual cycle and may also occur among pill-takers. Any worsening of this condition has not been proved to be directly related to pill use.

Weight change. Weight change and bloating while on the pill can be expected in some women, but these conditions are also influenced by eating and nutritional patterns. Weight gain of 2–4 kg (4–9 lb) is not uncommon in some women on the pill, and can be helped by diet or other means. Bloating usually occurs late in the menstrual cycle and is caused by increased water retention. Reduction of salt intake late in the cycle should help relieve this condition.

Libido change. Certainly nothing is more subjective in most people's lives than sex drive. Changes in libido among pill users can be affected by the normal uncertainties of daily life and are extremely difficult to measure in a clinical study. Pill users make frequent visits to clinics and are more aware of being monitored than are nonusers. Consequently, pill users may have more reasons and opportunities for reporting changes in their libido. A decrease in libido is sometimes reported among pill users, but these findings are subject to substantial bias. Several studies comparing the frequency of intercourse and orgasm in women before and after starting pill use found no differences in these measurements. There are even reports that some women experience an increased sex drive on the pill, perhaps because their fears of becoming pregnant have been relieved.

It is most important that the provider be familiar with both sets of possible side-effects occurring among women using the pill. These symptoms should always be treated with concern and understanding and reassurance or therapy provided where needed. An informed and confident clinician can prevent many minor problems from becoming more significant than necessary for the pill user.

Circulatory Complications

There are also rare but potentially serious conditions that have been found to have statistical association with oral contraceptive use. These conditions include thrombophlebitis, thromboembolism, stroke, subarachnoid hemorrhage, heart attack, hypertension, benign liver tumors, and possibly gallstones (Table 2-11). The incidence of these complications varies significantly according to the pill user's age and the presence of other disease risk factors—particularly cigarette smoking. Health practitioners providing oral contraceptives must be familiar with this variance in incidence. They also must be familiar with the symptoms of pill-associated complications and how to manage them. Both provider and client, however, should realize how rare these complications are when the client is properly screened. Any possible risks should also be weighed against the multiple benefits of pill use (see page 27).

Table 2-11. Complications of Oral Contraceptives.
• Thromboembolism • Thrombophlebitis • Stroke • Subarachnoid hemorrhage • Heart attack • Hypertension • Benign liver tumors • Gallstones

Introduction. The first serious complications discovered with pill use were circulatory, and they remain the area of greatest concern and attention. Beginning in the late 1960s, research focused on thrombophlebitis and thromboembolism. Today the focus has shifted to myocardial infarction and subarachnoid hemorrhage. What is as true today as it was 15 years ago is the epidemiological confusion and contradiction surrounding the exact nature of the increased risk of circulatory disease in pill users. This confusion remains despite oral contraceptives being the most intensively studied drug in history.

The only conclusion reached by all major studies on this subject is that tobacco smoking is a serious cause of circulatory disease, especially in older pill users (over 35 years of age). Some studies have documented significant circulatory disease risks only among pill users who smoke. Perhaps this association should be stated in the reverse of the usual warning: the harmful effects of smoking are intensified by pill use, rather than saying that pill use is especially dangerous if the woman smokes.

The major studies. Three large prospective studies are cited in this section: the RCGP study, the Oxford–FPA study, and the Walnut Creek study (Table 2-12). In this context, the term *prospective* means that the researchers followed the women forward through time from when they began pill-taking. This is the best epidemiological means of determining a drug's side-effects. Much of the popular and professional confusion has come from *retrospective* studies that find women with a certain disease and work "backward" to determine the proportion who used the pill. For many reasons, this approach is less useful than prospective studies.

The RCGP study began in the United Kingdom in 1968 and by 1981 had accumulated 184,000 woman-years of documented pill use. (Total woman-years is the total number of calendar months all study participants used the contraceptive method, divided by 12.) Another British study, sponsored by Oxford University and the British Family Planning Association (Oxford–FPA) began at the same time and by 1981 covered 80,000 woman-years of pill use. These two ongoing studies rely on clinicians' reports of side-effects and complications. The Walnut Creek study, which has followed more than 16,000 women in California for a decade, bases its findings on *hospitalization* rates for pill-related conditions.

Although these three studies sometimes differ in their conclusions, their size, length, and quality make them the best source of

Table 2-12.
Complications of Pill Use: Summary of Major Research Findings.

Complication	Study				
	RCGP	Walnut Creek	Oxford–FPA	BCDSP	Emory U.
Thrombosis	Y	N*			
Pulmonary embolism	N†	Y			
Thrombophlebitis		Y			
Stroke	N†	N*		Y	
Arterial embolism		N*			
Subarachnoid hemorrhage	?	Y	N		
Heart attack	Y/N*	N			
Significant hypertension		Y			N
Gallstones	N	N	N	Y	
Benign liver tumors†					

*Among nonsmokers.
†Too rare to study.
Y = positive association, ? = uncertain, N = not associated.

information from which to draw conclusions for clinical practice. Much of what follows is epidemiological, but the clinician should remember that risk factors and potential benefits must be balanced individually for each client. Therefore, clinical guidelines and warning symptoms are also included below.

Overall mortality risks. In an interim report, the RCGP study found that pill users had a five times greater risk of mortality from circulatory diseases than do never-users (26.8 versus 5.5 deaths per 100,000 woman-years, respectively). Similar findings of lesser magnitude have been found in other studies. On more detailed analysis covering more years of use, the RCGP now concludes that this increased mortality risk is almost entirely concentrated in pill users who smoke and who are over 35 years of age. For nonsmoking pill users under age 35, the risk of mortality and indeed most circulatory complications is apparently very low.

Data from the U.S. National Institute of Child Health and Human Development (NICHD) are shown in Table 2-13 and Figure 2-9. In terms of mortality from cardiovascular disease, use of oral contraceptives or other contraceptive methods by nonsmokers under age 35 is much safer than pregnancy. For smoking pill users 30–35

Table 2-13. Mortality in Pill Users by Age and Smoking Status.				
Age	Pregnancy	Nonsmoking Users of Other Contraceptive Methods	Nonsmoking Pill Users	Smoking Pill Users
15–19	4	1	1	2
30–34	15	3	3	12
40–44	21	2–5	18	61

Adapted from Stadel, 1981.
Risk in United States of cardiovascular mortality per 100,000 births per year or per 100,000 method users per year.

years old, risks are comparable to those encountered in pregnancy. This pattern changes for women over 40. Mortality for nonsmoking pill users rises to a level comparable to the risk from pregnancy, whereas the risk from using other methods remain very low. For *smoking* pill users over 40, the risk of mortality from cardiovascular disease is much greater. Despite the avalanche of disturbing statistics, therefore, the risk/benefit ratio for pill use in younger nonsmoking women is very favorable.

Several researchers have tried to determine the relationship between oral contraceptive use and circulatory disease by examining overall mortality statistics for a given population. These studies in the United Kingdom, United States, and Taiwan have all shown a *decline* in circulatory disease mortality for women since the introduction of the pill. Some family planning experts have asked, "Where are the deaths?" On the other hand, it has been pointed out that such an approach is a dubious means of drawing conclusions on the pill's safety. These statistics naturally report on older women, among whom the proportion of pill users is small. If they *had* been pill users, though, they probably had used pills with a high estrogen content. For now, the only conclusion that can be confidently drawn from these studies is that oral contraceptive use has not caused an increase in overall circulatory disease mortality.

Mechanism. At first only the estrogen component of the combined oral contraceptive pill was suspected as a cause of circulatory complications. This led to the sharp reduction in the pill's estrogen

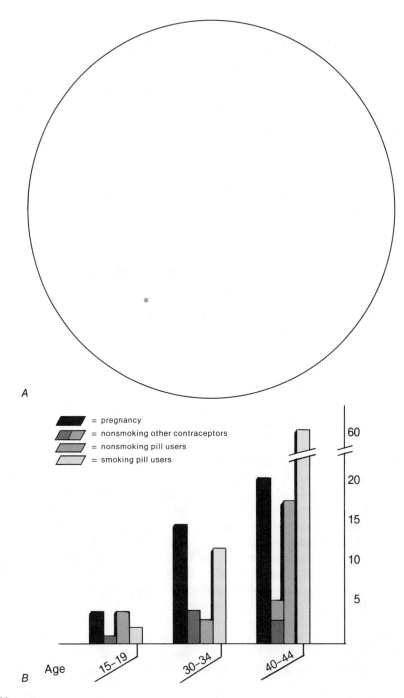

A

= pregnancy
= nonsmoking other contraceptors
= nonsmoking pill users
= smoking pill users

60
20
15
10
5

B Age   15–19   30–34   40–44

58

content and dictates the philosophy of choosing the lowest estrogen dose possible for each client. Subsequent research, however, has distinguished between *venous* and *arterial* complications. Venous complications involve clotting and include thrombophlebitis, thromboembolism, and thrombotic strokes. Arterial complications include hypertension, myocardial infarction, arterial occlusion, and subarachnoid hemorrhage.

Estrogen is generally blamed for venous complications, but the progestin component is now suspected for causing arterial complications. One study found that halving the amount of progestin reduced to half the already low incidence of myocardial infarction and stroke in pill users. As a result of these research findings, some experts now advise the clinician to seek the lowest possible progestin potency compatible with manageable and effective oral contraception. Table 2-7 shows the relative progestational potency of the commonly used progestin formulations.

Thrombophlebitis, thromboembolism, and stroke. The occurrence of thrombotic complications among oral contraceptive users is thought to be related to the estrogen content of the pill. The RCGP study found that *deep* vein thrombosis of the legs (which can lead to thromboembolism) occurred four times more often in pill users than nonusers. Superficial vein thrombosis (a far less serious condition) occurred two times more frequently among pill users. Apparently, the increased risk of thrombosis only occurs in current pill users, and disappears when pill use is discontinued.

The now classical association of pill use with thrombophlebitis and thromboembolism is being questioned by some researchers because of inconsistencies in individual clinician's diagnoses in earlier studies. For instance, the Walnut Creek study confirmed that pill users run a higher risk of pulmonary embolism and thrombophlebitis, but they did *not* find an increased risk of arterial embolism, thrombosis, cerebral hemorrhage or stroke among *nonsmoking* pill users.

A retrospective study by the Boston Collaborative Drug Surveillance Program (BCDSP) conducted in Washington State from 1977 to 1979, including 40,000 women, found that venous thromboembo-

Figure 2-9. *(A) Overall annual risk of cardiovascular mortality among nonsmoking pill users under 40 years of age—less than 3 per 100,000. (B) Mortality in pill users by age and smoking status; deaths per 100,000 births or method users per year. (Adapted from Stadel, 1981.)*

lism occurred eight times more frequently in oral contraceptive users than nonusers. Despite this increase, the incidence of thromboembolism in otherwise healthy pill users was estimated at 19 per 100,000 woman-years of use—a very low rate. The study did not control for smoking. No association was found between pill use and stroke. In the RCGP study, pulmonary embolism, cerebral hemorrhage, and cerebral thrombosis could not be studied at all despite the participation of 23,000 pill users because the number of reported episodes was so small.

The risk of thromboembolism is highest for women over age 40 and for those who smoke heavily. This risk does not rise with duration of pill use (except as age increases), and there is no evidence that an excess risk of thromboembolism persists after pill use has been discontinued.

Overall, the "excess mortality" among pill users caused by thromboembolism has been estimated to be 1–3 deaths per 100,000 woman-years. During the more than 450,000 woman-years of pill use studied in the United Kingdom since 1968, only 5 mortalities associated with venous thromboembolic disease have been reported.

The clinician should be aware that thromboembolism and stroke are often preceded by ample warning, such as thrombophlebitis or severe headache. Any thrombotic or embolic complications with pill use demand immediate cessation of oral contraceptives. Awareness of the relationship of the pill to these conditions will further aid the clinician in prevention of any serious health hazard.

Subarachnoid hemorrhage.   Evidence is contradictory on the association of subarachnoid hemorrhage with oral contraceptive use. A subarachnoid hemorrhage results from the rupture of a weak blood vessel of the brain. An interim RCGP report found an increased risk of mortality from this condition among pill users. The actual number of deaths in the study from subarachnoid hemorrhage among pill users was small, and the results are subject to possible errors in diagnosis and interpretation. Since no deaths from subarachnoid hemorrhage occurred in women not taking the pill, the data did therefore suggest an increased risk of this condition that may linger after the pill has been discontinued. The Walnut Creek study confirmed this conclusion, finding the association to exist independently of smoking habits.

The Oxford–FPA study, however, has *not* found an association between pill use and subarachnoid hemorrhage. Their conclusion is that hypertension may be the risk factor, not pill use.

Heart attack (myocardial infarction). The development of heart attack does not appear to be specifically related to the estrogen content in oral contraceptives. Rather, it is more likely related to the balance of the estrogen and progestin in the pill and their effects on the lipids (fats) in the blood. The RCGP study at first confirmed that the risk of death from heart attack was three times greater for women using the pill than for nonusers (8.1 versus 2.5 deaths per 100,000 woman-years). The most recent RCGP data indicate that the mortality risk from heart attack is concentrated in older pill users who smoke. The Walnut Creek study did not find myocardial infarction to be associated with pill use, but rather *only* with smoking. The BCDSP–Washington study found no cases of myocardial infarction in over 36,000 woman-years of pill use.

A 1981 retrospective study of myocardial infarction was the first to find that the increased risk of heart attack among oral contraceptive users may persist after the woman stops taking the pill. This study found an overall increased risk of myocardial infarction of 3.5 times for current pill users compared to nonusers. For former users who had taken the pill for 10 years or more, the relative risk was still high—2.5 (although less for women who had used the pill for less time). No other study has yet duplicated these findings. One possible explanation for this finding is that women who had used the pill for 10 or more years had probably used pills containing much larger doses of estrogen than those normally used today. The RCGP study has not been able to study this residual effect in past users because the total number of heart attack cases has been so small. They have *not* found the risk of myocardial infarction to increase with duration of pill use among ever users.

The occurrence of heart attack among pill users appears to be associated with a number of predisposing risk factors, including cigarette smoking, age, obesity, diabetes, and hypertension. Several predisposing risk factors for heart attack may exist at the same time, and it is difficult to determine the precise significance of each risk factor for any individual pill user. Nevertheless, the effects of these factors seem to be additive with the exception of cigarette smoking, which appears to have a synergistic (greater than additive) effect with the pill on the risk of heart attack. In fact, a British study found that heavy cigarette smoking (over 25 cigarettes a day) was more likely to lead to heart attack than was oral contraceptive use. Data from studies in the United States and Great Britain indicate that nonsmoking pill users under age 40 have a 50% (1.5 times) greater risk of mortality from myocardial infarction than nonsmoking nonusers, but the risk is still very low (1.8 versus 1.2 deaths per 100,000 woman-years). *Smoking* pill users under 40, however, have an *eight* times greater risk of death from heart attack (see Table 2-13 and Figure 2-9B).

Risk guidelines. In view of the above research findings, it is recommended that family planning providers strongly discourage the practice of cigarette smoking among all pill users. The following general guidelines may assist family planning providers to reduce the possibility of circulatory disease among oral contraceptive users:

1. Women under age 35 who take the pill should be advised to refrain from cigarette smoking.
2. Women aged 35–39 who have conditions predisposing to circulatory system disease (smoking, obesity, diabetes, hypertension) should not take the pill unless no alternative contraceptive method is acceptable, or if the maternal health risks of pregnancy are excessive. For many of these women, an effective long-term contraceptive alternative is the IUD. Condoms or diaphragm backed up by freely available therapeutic abortion in case of contraceptive failure can also be a practical alternative.
3. Women over age 40 should not use oral contraceptives if at all possible. However, in those countries where the pill is the only available effective contraceptive and pregnancy is dangerous, use of oral contraceptives may still be the "better" risk. In addition to other contraceptive methods, voluntary sterilization may be highly satisfactory for couples in this age group.

Developing countries. In most developing countries, relatively few women are cigarette smokers. Only 15% of oral contraceptive users in most family planning programs are over age 35. The incidence of other conditions predisposing to circulatory disease is also low (with the exception of hypertension in some areas), as are the actual disease rates. One researcher has calculated that the prevalence in a developing country population of risk factors leading to heart attack may be only 19% of the prevalence of these factors in developed countries. The study projected the occurrence of 4 deaths

---

Figure 2-10. *Risks of contraception and maternity in developed (A) and developing (B) countries; deaths per 100,000 births or method users per year. (Adapted from Potts et al., 1978.)*

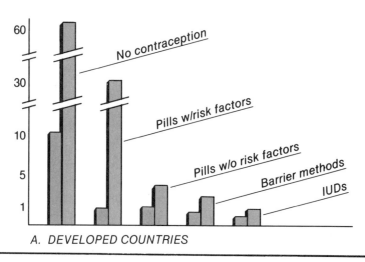

A. DEVELOPED COUNTRIES

B. DEVELOPING COUNTRIES, RURAL AREAS

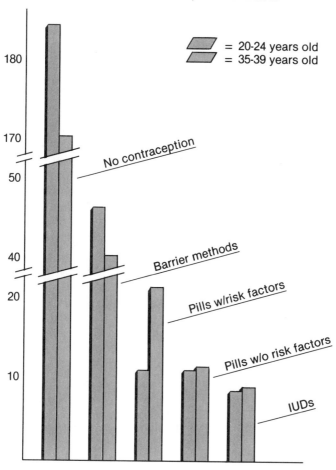

= 20-24 years old
= 35-39 years old

from myocardial infarction per *one million* pill users annually in a developing country.

The risks of contraception must be compared to the benefits—the protection from certain diseases and the prevention of the risks from the unwanted pregnancy that may otherwise occur. The risk of death from pregnancy and childbirth in some areas of developing countries is staggering and tragic—as high as 700 per 100,000 live births, or almost 1 in 100. Rates of 300 or more are not uncommon. To place the risks of pill use in this perspective, the International Fertility Research Program (IFRP) prepared risk estimates for maternity and contraceptive use in three settings—developed countries, advanced urban areas in developing countries, and poorer rural developing country settings. The risk estimates shown in Figure 2-10 convincingly demonstrate the danger of maternity—a needless risk when pregnancy is unwanted.

Hypertension. The meaning of the term *hypertension* is highly variable. In studying the relationship between hypertension and oral contraceptive use, researchers have distinguished *mild* hypertension from *clinical* or *significant* hypertension. Arbitrarily setting a worldwide standard of significant hypertension is not useful, and even when definitions are agreed on, large clinical studies have produced conflicting conclusions on incidence. It does appear that a majority of pill users experience a *mild* increase in blood pressure while on oral contraceptives. Their blood pressure almost always returns to preexisting levels after pill use is discontinued.

Some women may develop *significant* hypertension during pill use, although this is usually due to predisposing factors. The Walnut Creek study at first found the incidence of significant hypertension (defined by the study as blood pressure over 140/90) to be 4% in pill users compared to 1.5% in nonusers, but the most recent report found a lower risk differential. A study at Emory University in Atlanta, involving 20,000 black pill-takers, did *not* find an association between pill use and significant hypertension, and yet blacks are known to be particularly susceptible to high blood pressure.

If significant hypertension is confirmed in a woman on oral contraceptives, the patient should be identified as requiring further medical evaluation. If this condition is persistent, oral contraceptives should be stopped promptly. Blood pressure generally returns to normal in women with pill-revealed hypertension after they stop taking the pill. By itself, mild hypertension in pill users does not require special treatment. Considering the role of hypertension in

cardiovascular disease, however, and the relationship of oral contraceptive use with myocardial infarction, women already at a high
risk because of *other predisposing factors* such as smoking, obesity,
and diabetes should consider another method of contraception, if
available. In evaluating the health risk of mild hypertension in pill
users, the clinician and the patient should remember that the unwanted pregnancy that can result from less effective contraception
can also induce elevated blood pressure.

Because of the possible increase in hypertension observed with
pill use, it has been suggested by some practitioners that all women
should stop oral contraceptive use every 2 years or so to prevent the
development of hypertensive problems. The RCGP study found no
evidence that stopping pill use periodically is beneficial to the patient. Instead, the study found an unwanted pregnancy rate of 20
per 100 woman-years among those women who stopped taking the
pill. Thus, temporary pill discontinuation exposes patients to possible unwanted pregnancy without clinical justification.

Other Complications

Benign liver tumors (hepatic adenoma). The extremely rare
condition of benign liver tumor (hepatic adenoma) has been reported among oral contraceptive users. The total number of cases
reported thus far is so low that a rate of incidence cannot be estimated. There is no known way that the formation of liver tumors
can be predicted or prevented, and neither is there any practical
method of early detection. Almost all these rare pill-associated cases
have been reported among long-term pill users.

Benign liver tumors occur in women who do not take the pill, of
course, but it appears that if they develop in pill users, they are
more likely to be associated with rupture and significant bleeding.
Any oral contraceptive user with an enlarged liver, abdominal pain,
or findings suggestive of intraabdominal bleeding requires immediate medical evaluation.

Gallstones (cholelithiasis). The previously assumed connection
between oral contraceptive use and gallbladder disease is now being
questioned. The Boston study (BCDSP) found evidence of a relationship between oral contraceptive use and gallstones (cholelithiasis).
This study found gallstones twice as often in pill users as in nonusers, occurring at an approximate rate of 60 cases per 100,000 pill
users per year. A relationship of oral contraceptives and gallstones

was confirmed in the RCGP study but was not found to be statistically significant. The Walnut Creek study did not reveal an association between pill use and gallbladder disease, and neither did a review of Oxford–FPA data performed by the CDC. At first, a relationship between oral contraceptives and gallstones was confirmed by the RCGP study. But now that study, along with the CDC review, concludes that oral contraceptives are *not* an important risk factor in the development of gallbladder disease, but they may *uncover* those women prone to the condition. This will usually occur within the first 6 months of pill use, enabling the clinician to quickly evaluate and treat the condition. Pill use should be discontinued when gallstones are found.

Other Metabolic Effects

Other areas of concern about oral contraceptive use include the potential changes in metabolism and the nutritional status in some pill-takers. Oral contraceptives have been found to affect chemical processes in the liver and to slightly alter the levels of some chemical substances circulating in the blood. These changes do not have major effects on health, and their physiological significance is questionable.

Similarly, there have been reports of various vitamin and trace mineral deficiencies—particularly folic acid and also pyridoxine (vitamin B_6)—which may be associated with oral contraceptive use. The clinical significance of any pill-related deficiencies of these substances is small and is particularly variable depending on local nutrition. No precaution need be taken other than to observe oral contraceptive users for any possible nutritional deficiencies according to standard public health practice. Should such deficiencies become evident, they can be corrected by vitamin supplementation or nutritional counseling.

A recent study has found that long-term oral contraceptive use may increase the effect of the common tranquilizer diazepam (Valium). When prescribing diazepam, physicians should check on the client's contraceptive use and consider lowering the diazepam dosage for oral contraceptive users.

Subsequent Fertility

Prospective and current users of oral contraceptives commonly have serious concerns about their subsequent fertility after discontinuing pill use. These concerns are unnecessary since oral contraceptives have not been found to increase or decrease fertility. Providers should carefully correct any client misconceptions about the information that follows.

In general, women who attempt conception after stopping pill use will take a few months longer to become pregnant than will women just stopping the use of other contraceptive methods. A 1982 report concluded that the chance of conception in former pill takers is particularly reduced within the first 3 months after discontinuing use. In another study that concentrated on *ovulation*, not conception, 85% of the women tested ovulated within 6 weeks of stopping pill use. This compares favorably to the normal postpartum experience in women not breastfeeding.

There may sometimes be a delay in the resumption of regular menstruation (temporary amenorrhea) after pills are discontinued, but this condition lasts only a few weeks in most cases. Studies indicate that the rare occurrence of prolonged postpill amenorrhea is usually related to underlying preexisting menstrual dysfunction rather than the pill itself. Patients will rarely need medical treatment for amenorrhea following oral contraceptive use, and should be given appropriate reassurance in the interim.

Fears about the effects on children born to women who have previously taken the pill are unfounded. No research has found that the pill has any adverse effects on the course and outcome of *subsequent* pregnancies or that there is an increase of congenital abnormalities among children of former pill-takers as compared to controls. Studies have also shown no effect of previous pill use on the course of subsequent pregnancy and labor.

Some studies have suggested that children born to women who inadvertently *continue* oral contraceptives during the early pregnancy may have a slightly higher incidence of congenital abnormalities. For this reason, users of oral contraceptives should immediately discontinue the pill if pregnancy is diagnosed or strongly suspected. As an added precaution, some clinicians recommend that oral contraceptive users who wish to become pregnant should stop the pill and use an alternative contraceptive method for a month or two to reduce the possibility of any lingering deleterious effects from the pill. This may be unnecessary, however: a World Health Organization (WHO) Scientific Group concluded in a 1981 report that even in cases of inadvertent overlap of pill use and early pregnancy, the risk of effects on the fetus is too low to estimate.

CONCLUSION

Although this chapter has focused on oral contraceptives, in general it is undesirable to emphasize only one method of contraception in family planning service. Other effective methods are discussed in the remaining chapters of this book. Each individual will prefer to have the opportunity to choose among a variety of different methods, and the offering of a broad choice will result in broad acceptance. In addition, since not every method is medically suitable for every client, offering different contraceptive techniques is essential for safe clinical practice.

The reader may feel overwhelmed by this chapter's detailed discussion of possible side-effects and complications from oral contraceptive use. In closing it is important to emphasize that the great majority of pill users will experience none of the side-effects described here after the first few months of use and that the occurrence of serious complications from pill use is rare. The risk of incurring any one of the major complications is less than 1 in 1000, and the risk of subsequent mortality is even rarer.

As an overview of the balance between the pill's advantages and disadvantages, the RCGP conclusion is particularly relevant: "The estimated risk at the present time of using the pill is one that a properly informed woman would be happy to take."

Selected Readings

Abernathy DR, Greenblatt DJ, Divoll M, et al: Impairment of diazepam metabolism by low-dose estrogen-containing oral contraceptive steroids. New England Journal of Medicine 306(13): 791, April 1, 1982.

Adam SA, Sheaves JK, Wright NH, et al: A case-control study of the possible association between oral contraceptives and malignant melanoma. British Journal of Cancer 44: 45, 1981

Adam SA, Thorogood M, Mann JI; Oral contraception and myocardial infarction revisited: Effects of new preparations and prescribing patterns. British Journal of Obstetrics and Gynecology 99: 838, 1981

Anonymous: Children of pill users who breastfeed show no growth deficiencies. International Family Planning Perspectives 8(1): 30, March 1982

Anonymous: Method for quick, accurate headache evaluations. Contraceptive Technology Update 1(3): 45, June 1980

Atkinson L, Castadot R, Cuadros A, Rosenfeld AG: Oral contraceptives: Considerations of safety in nonclinical distribution. Studies in Family Planning 5(8): 242, August 1974

Bader M: Oral contraceptives and myocardial infarction. New England Journal of Medicine 297(8): 449, May 19, 1977

Belsey MA: The risks and benefits of oral contraceptives in the developing world. Acta Obstetricia et Gynecologica Scandinavica Suppl. 105: 61, 1982

Boyce JG, Lu T, Nelson JH, Fruchter RG: Oral contraceptives and cervical carcinoma. American Journal of Obstetrics and Gynecology 128(7): 761, August 1, 1977

Briggs MH, Briggs M: Oral Contraceptives. Eden Press Annual Research Reviews, vol. 5. Westmount, Quebec, Eden Press, 1981, 331 pp

Bromwich PD, Parsons AD: The establishment of a postcoital contraception service. The British Journal of Family Planning 8: 16, 1982

Chow L, Nair N: Oral contraceptive use and diseases of the circulatory system in Taiwan: An analysis of mortality statistics. International Journal of Gynecology and Obstetrics 18(6): 420, 1980

Collaborative Group for the Study of Stroke in Young Women: Oral contraceptives and stroke in young women: Associated risk factors. Journal of the American Medical Association 231(7): 718, February 17, 1975

Cook RJ: Distribution of oral contraceptives: Legal changes and new concepts of preventive care. American Journal of Public Health 66(6): 590, June 1976

Cramer DW, Hutchison GB, Welch WR, et al: Factors affecting the association of oral contraceptives and ovarian cancer. New England Journal of Medicine 307(17): 1047, October 21, 1982

Dickey RP: Initial pill selection and managing the contraceptive pill patient. International Journal of Gynecology and Obstetrics 16(6): 547, 1979

Fasal E, Paffenberger RS: Oral contraceptives as related to cancer and benign lesions of breast. Journal of the National Cancer Institute 55: 767, October 1975

Fisch IR, Frank J: Oral contraceptives and blood pressure. Journal of American Medical Association 237(23): 2499, June 6, 1977

Goldzieher J: Oral contraceptive hazards—1981. Fertility and Sterility 35(3): 275, March 1981

Guillebaud J: Missed pills—what advice should we give? The British Journal of Family Planning 7(2): 41, July 1981

Heiby JR: The association of oral contraceptives and myocardial infarction in less-developed countries, in Sciarra JJ, Zatuchni GI, Speidel JJ (eds): Risks, Benefits and Controversies in Fertility Control. Hagerstown, MD, Harper & Row, 1978, p 162

Huber DH, Huber SC: Screening oral contraceptive candidates and inconsequential pelvic examinations. Studies in Family Planning 6(2): 49, February 1975

Huggins GR, Fiuntoli RL: Oral contraceptives and neoplasia. Fertility and Sterility 32(1): 1, July 1979

Hulka BS, Chambless LE, Kaufman DG, et al: Protection against endometrial carcinoma by combination-product oral contraceptives. Journal of the American Medical Association 247(4): 475, January 22/29, 1982

Hull MG, Bromham DR, Savage PE, et al: Normal fertility in women with post-pill amenorrhoea. Lancet 1: 1329, June 20, 1981

Inman WHW: Oral contraceptives and fatal subarachnoid hemorrhage. British Medical Journal 2: 468, 1979

Inman WHW, Vessey MP, Esterholm B, et al: Thromboembolic disease and the steroidal content of oral contraceptives: A report to the Committee on Safety of Drugs. British Medical Journal 2: 203, 1970

Jain AK: Cigarette smoking, use of oral contraceptives, and myocardial infarction. American Journal of Obstetrics and Gynecology 126(3): 301, October 1, 1976

Jain AK: Mortality risk associated with the use of oral contraceptives. Studies in Family Planning 8(3): 50, March 1977

Janerich DT, Piper JM: Epidemiologic studies on the effect of oral contraceptives on subsequent pregnancies, in Sciarra JJ, Zatuchni GI, Speidel JJ (eds): Risks, Benefits and Controversies in Fertility Control. Hagerstown, MD, Harper & Row, 1978, p 263

Jick H, Dinan B, Rothman KJ: Oral contraceptives and nonfatal myocardial infarction. Journal of American Medical Association 239(14): 1403, April 3, 1978

Kols A, Rinehart W, Piotrow PT, et al: Oral contraceptives in the 1980s. Population Reports A(6), Baltimore, Johns Hopkins University, May/June 1982

Lahteenmaki P, Ylostalo P, Sipinen S, et al: Return of ovulation after abortion and after discontinuation of oral contraceptives. Fertility and Sterility 34(3): 246, September 1980

Laragh JH: Oral contraceptives-induced hypertension: Nine years later. American Journal of Obstetrics and Gynecology 126(1): 141, September 1, 1976

Larsson-Cohn U: Oral contraceptives and vitamins: A review. American Journal of Obstetrics and Gynecology 121(1): 84, January 1, 1975

Law B: Advantages and disadvantages of low-dose oral contraceptives. International Journal of Gynecology and Obstetrics 16(6): 556, 1979

Layde PM, Beral V: Further analyses of mortality in oral contraceptive users. Lancet 1: 541, March 7, 1981

Layde PM, Ory HW, Schlesselman JJ: The risk of myocardial infarction in former users of oral contraceptives. Family Planning Perspectives 14(2): 78, March/April 1982

Linn S, Schoenbaum SC, Monson RR, et al: Delay in conception for former pill users. Journal of the American Medical Association 247(5): 629, February 5, 1982

Mann JI, Vessey MP: Trends in cardiovascular disease mortality and oral contraceptives. The British Journal of Family Planning 6: 99, 1981

Nissen ED, Kent DR, Nissen SE, et al: Association of liver tumors with oral contraceptives. Obstetrics and Gynecology 48(1): 49, July 1976

Nora JJ, Nora AA: Can the pill cause birth defects? New England Journal of Medicine 291(14): 731, October 3, 1974

Oakley N. Stanton SL: Contraception and diabetes. British Journal of Family Planning 8: 55, 1982

Ortiz-Perez HE, Fuertes-de la Haba A, Bangdiwala IS, et al: Abnormalities among offspring of oral and nonoral contraceptive users. American Journal of Obstetrics and Gynecology 134(5): 512, July 1, 1979

Ory H, Cole p, MacMahon B, Hoover R: Oral contraceptives and reduced risk of benign breast disease. New England Journal of Medicine 294(8): 419, February 19, 1976

Ory H, Naib Z, Conger SB, et al: Contraceptive choice and prevalence of cervical dysplasia and carcinoma in situ. American Journal of Obstetrics and Gynecology 124(6): 573, March 15, 1976

Ory HW, Rosenfield A, Landman LC: The pill at 20: An assessment. Family Planning Perspectives 12: 278, November/December 1980

Petitti DB, Wingerd J: Use of oral contraceptives, cigarette smoking, and risk of subarachnoid hemorrhage. Lancet 2: 234, July 29, 1978

Porter JB, Hunter JR, Danielson DA, et al: Oral contraceptives and nonfatal vascular disease—recent experience. Obstetrics and Gynecology 59(3): 299, March 1982

Potts M, Speidel JJ, Kessel E: Relative risks of various means of fertility control when used in less-developed countries, in Sciarra JJ, Zatuchni GI, Speidel JJ (eds): Risks, Benefits and Controversies in Fertility Control. Hagerstown, MD, Harper & Row, 1978, p 28

Rinehart W, Piotrow PT: Oral contraceptives—update on usage, safety and side-effects. Population Reports A(5). Baltimore, Population Information Program, January 1979, 53 pp

Rothman KJ, Louik C: Oral contraceptives and birth defects. New England Journal of Medicine 299(10): 522, September 7, 1978

Rowlands S, Guillebaud J: Postcoital contraception. The British Journal of Family Planning 7: 3, April 1981

Royal College of General Practitioners; Oral contraceptives and health—an interim report. New York, Pitman, 1974, 98 pp

Royal College of General Practitioners: Mortality among oral contraceptive users. Lancet 2: 727, October 8, 1977

Royal College of General Practitioners: Reduction in incidence of rheumatoid arthritis associated with oral contraceptives. Lancet 1: 569, March 18, 1978

Royal College of General Practitioners: Further analyses of mortality in oral contraceptive users. Lancet 1: 541, March 7, 1981

Sartwell PE, Masi AT, Arthes FG, et al: Thromboembolism and oral contraceptives: An epidemiologic case-control study. American Journal of Epidemiology 90(5): 365, 1969

Senanayake P, Kramer DG: Contraception and pelvic inflammatory disease. IPPF Medical Bulletin 16(2): 3, April 1982

Shapiro S. Slone S, Rosenberg L, et al: Oral contraceptive use in relation to myocardial infarction. Lancet 1: 743, April 7, 1979

Silverberg SG, Makowski EL: Endometrial carcinoma in young women taking oral contraceptives. Obstetrics and Gynecology 46(5): 503, November 1975

Slone D, Shapiro S, et al: Risk of myocardial infarction in relation to current and discontinued use of oral contraceptives. New England Journal of Medicine 305(8): 420, August 20, 1981

Spellacy WN, Wynn V, (eds): Progestogens and the cardiovascular system. American Journal of Obstetrics and Gynecology 142(6): 717, part 2, March 15, 1982

Stadel BV: Oral contraceptives and cardiovascular disease, Part I. New England Journal of Medicine 305(11): 612, September 10, 1981

Stadel, BV: Oral contraceptives and cardiovascular disease, Part II. New England Journal of Medicine 305(12): 672, September 17, 1981

Stern E, Forsythe AB, Youkeles L, Coffelt CF: Steroid contraceptive use and cervical dysplasia: Increased risk of progression. Science 196: 1460, June 24, 1977

Swyer GIM: Potency of progestogens in oral contraceptives—further delay of menses data. Contraception 26(1): 23, July 1982

Taber BZ: Breast cancer and oral contraceptives. Journal of Reproductive Medicine 15(3): 97, September 1979

Thorogood M, et al: Fatal subanachnoid hemorrhage in young women: role of oral contraceptives. British Medical Journal 283: 762, September 19, 1981

Tieng P, Gray RH: The return of fertility following discontinuation of oral contraceptives in Thailand. Fertility and Sterility 35(5): 532, May 1981

Tietze C: The pill and mortality from cardiovascular disease: Another look. Family Planning Perspectives 11(2): 80, March/April 1979

Tietze C, Lewit S: Life risk associated with reversible methods of fertility regulation. International Journal of Gynecology and Obstetrics 16(6): 456, 1979

Van Campenhout J, Blanchet P, Beauregard H, et al: Amenorrhea following the use of oral contraceptives. Fertility and Sterility 28(7): 728, July 1977

Vana J, Murphy GP, Aronoff BL, et al: Primary liver tumors and oral contraceptives: Results of survey. Journal of the American Medical Association 238(20): 2154, November 14, 1977

Vandenbroucke JP, Valkenberg HA, Boersma JW, et al: Oral contraceptives and rheumatoid arthritis: Further evidence for a preventive effect. Lancet 2:839, October 16, 1982

Vessey MP, Doll R, Jones K, et al: An epidemiological study of oral contraceptives and breast cancer. British Medical Journal 1: 1757, 1979

Vessey MP, Lawless M, Yeates D: Efficacy of different contraceptive methods. Lancet 1:841, April 10, 1982

Vessey MP, McPherson K, Johnson B: Mortality among women participating in the Oxford/Family Planning Association contraceptive study. Lancet 2: 731, October 8, 1977

Vessey MP, McPherson K, Yeates D: Mortality in oral contraceptive users. Lancet 1: 549, March 7, 1981

Vessey MP, Meisler L, Flavel R, Yeates D: Outcome of pregnancy in women using different methods of contraception. British Journal of Obstetrics and Gynecology 86: 548, 1979

Vessey MP, Wright NH, McPherson K, et al: Fertility after stopping different methods of contraception. British Medical Journal 1: 265, February 4, 1978

Viravaidya M: Nonphysicians in family planning and family health in Thailand, in Waife RS, Burkhart MC, eds: The Nonphysician and Family Health in Sub-Sahara Africa. Chestnut Hill, MA, The Pathfinder Fund, 1981, p 71

Walnut Creek Contraceptive Drug Study: The Journal of Reproductive Medicine 25(6) (supplement): 349, December 1980

Williams R, Neuberger J: Occurrence, frequency and management of oral contraceptive associated liver tumors. British Journal of Family Planning 7(2): 35, July 1981

Wiseman, RA, MacRae KD: Oral contraceptives and the decline in mortality from circulatory disease. Fertility and Sterility 35(3): 277, March, 1981

World Health Organization: The effect of female sex hormones on fetal development and infant health. WHO Technical Report Series No. 657, 1981

Wortman J: Training nonphysicians in family planning services. Population Reports J(6), Washington, DC, George Washington University, September 1975

Yuzpe AA, Smith RP, Rademaker AW: A multicenter clinical investigation employing ethinyl estradiol combined with dl-norgestrel as a postcoital contraceptive agent. Fertility and Sterility 37(4): 508, April 1982

Intrauterine Devices

3

For centuries, people have sought a safe method of preventing pregnancy that is not directly tied to the act of sexual intercourse, that provides complete protection for as long as it is used, does not require regular attention, and whose effect is readily reversible. The intrauterine device (IUD) was designed to approach this goal. Once an IUD is inserted into a woman's uterus, it remains highly effective in preventing pregnancy for as long as it is in place. The frequency of side-effects in some women, however, has left the IUD short of the ideal.

Approximately 15 million women around the world are now using an IUD. Despite the widespread use of IUDs, there has been a good deal of confusion about their safety and proper role in family planning services. This confusion can in part be traced to the numerous different types of IUDs—loops, coils, spirals, shields, springs, and rings—that have been developed over the years. Some devices have been failures, while others have been very successful. The Lippes Loop, one of the first flexible plastic IUDS, still has the best established record of performance. The Saf-T-Coil (double coil) device has also been proven to be useful. The Dalkon Shield was popular before it was discontinued because of its association with infected spontaneous abortions among women who became pregnant with the shield in place (see page 116). Now the copper-releasing IUDs, specifically the Copper T and Copper 7 (Gravigard) and Multiload Cu250, are frequently chosen for contraception.

In theory, IUDs are an ideal contraceptive because:

- They are nearly 100% effective.
- They require only one insertion for prolonged protection.
- Their contraceptive effect is not directly related to each act of intercourse.
- Their contraceptive effect is readily reversible.

Recently, however, there has been serious concern about the morbidity associated with intrauterine devices, raising legitimate doubts about reliance on IUDs as a contraceptive method. These reports merit careful consideration but have tended to overemphasize the hazards and ignore the benefits of IUDs. For selected women, especially those who have had several pregnancies (multiparas), IUDs continue to be a useful family planning choice.

HISTORY

It is often reported that the first IUDs were small stones placed by desert nomads in the uteri of their camels in order to prevent pregnancies during long caravan journeys. In humans, the historical development of IUDs can be traced from the use of pessaries (instruments for supporting or occluding the uterus). Vaginal pessaries have been used for a multitude of gynecological conditions, and some were designed to have a contraceptive effect. As early as the 11th century, the Islamic scientist Avicenna described a pessary of pulp, mandrake root, sulfur, and tar to be "worn" after menstruation to prevent pregnancy. In the 19th century, metal pessaries were used that had stems that protruded through the cervical canal and into the uterine cavity. But none of these early devices were technically intrauterine—they did not rest entirely inside the uterus.

The first true IUD—a ring of silkworm gut string—was reported by Richter in 1909 in a German medical journal (Figure 3-1). The two most well-known IUDs before the 1960s were the Grafenberg rings of silver invented in Germany and the Ota rings of reinforced gold-plated silver invented in Japan. Although both the Grafenberg and Ota rings were successful in preventing pregnancies, many physicians condemned them for a variety of reasons, both theoretical and clinical, and their use was infrequent after the middle 1930s. Their effectiveness and safety were again documented in the late 1950s.

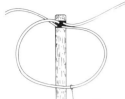

Figure 3-1. *An early IUD: ring of silkworm gut.*

A revolution in IUD technology occurred in the early 1960s with the development of biologically safe plastics. These new materials permitted the design of IUDs that were easily pliable, with a "memory" that enabled a device to return to its original shape after being compressed or stretched. Thus plastic IUDs could be designed that fit through inserter tubes of small diameter, minimizing cervical dilation and significantly increasing the safety of the insertion procedure. Bleeding and pain were found to be much less frequent with the plastic devices compared to the rigid metal designs, whereas contraceptive effectiveness remained high. The Lippes Loop was the first plastic IUD to be widely successful and today remains the worldwide "standard" against which the effectiveness and safety of all IUDs are measured.

The next major IUD breakthrough came in the late 1960s, when researchers began to wrap plastic devices with copper wire. Zipper, working in Chile, found that the release of copper ions into the uterine cavity increased the contraceptive effectiveness of IUDs. The copper devices, especially the "T" and "7" shapes, have been highly successful. They are generally smaller than the earlier IUDs and can achieve a level of safety and efficacy previously only possible with larger devices. The major drawback of the copper IUDs is that at present they must be changed every 3 or 4 years, but this inconvenience is balanced by their low level of side-effects and high effectiveness. Many other devices have been developed including those that release tiny amounts of a progestational hormones through the plastic in an attempt to improve efficacy and physiological tolerance.

EFFECTIVENESS AND EFFECTS

In theory, IUDs are second to "the pill" as a reliable means of reversible contraception, with an estimated failure rate of 1%–3%. Oral contraceptives do have a slightly higher rate of theoretical effectiveness (less than 1% failure rate) when taken consistently and correctly, but when contraceptive effectiveness is studied in actual use, IUDs sometimes can be superior to the pill (see Figure 2-1).

Since women using oral contraceptives must remember to take a pill daily, they must also be continually motivated to do so. Use of an IUD, on the other hand, does not require conscious effort on a day-to-day basis. Thus *continuing* use is often better with IUDs than with oral contraceptives. For example, the Population Council's Co-operative Statistical Program (CSP) that received reports on thousands of IUD insertions from around the world found in 1970 than an average of only 23% of women using Lippes Loop size D stopped using it (for all reasons) within 1 year. In comparison, discontinuation rates in the first year among oral contraceptive users have ranged up to 50%.

Mortality and Morbidity

Both the IUD and the pill are recognized for their superior effectiveness over other contraceptive methods. They are, however, also associated with more side-effects than the barrier methods (condom, foam, or diaphragm). The risk of mortality from an IUD is less than that from oral contraceptives: under 1 death per 100,000 woman-years for IUD users, compared to an estimated 1–4 deaths per 100,000 woman-years among users of oral contraceptives under the age of 35 who do not smoke, according to latest studies.

Since the incidence of cardiovascular disease in all people rises with age, so does the mortality from pill use, reaching 18 per 100,000 woman-years for users aged 40–44 years who do not smoke, and higher for those who do. In comparison, the mortality risk from IUDs is the same for women of all ages (see Figure 2-10). In terms of mortality, therefore, IUDs are much safer than the pill (or pregnancy) for older women. The rare death associated with IUD use has been caused by infection usually related to spontaneous abortion, or by undiagnosed ectopic pregnancy (see page 117).

The risk of morbidity (nonfatal complications or disease) *requiring hospitalization* appears to be higher from IUD use than from oral contraceptive use, principally because of the risk of uterine perforation and pelvic infection. In both an absolute and relative sense, however, risk of significant morbidity or mortality from IUDs are small, especially compared with the medical and social risks of unwanted pregnancy. This is especially true for developing countries, where maternal mortality may be as high as 700 deaths per 100,000 live births. Thus an IUD can be many times safer for a woman than the unwanted pregnancy that might occur if she used less effective contraception or no contraception at all.

Evaluation

When different IUD designs are evaluated, the Lippes Loop has served as the basic yardstick of comparison. Evaluation of the different IUDs is not a simple matter, however, and must take into consideration a number of factors, including incidence of pregnancy, spontaneous expulsion rates, and removals for bleeding and pain. These "event rates" can serve as a statistical predictor of the success or failure of a particular device design. Interpretation of data collected from clinical trials is complicated by the fact that there may be great variation in results when the same device is studied at different clinical centers. The difference in event rates obtained by separate clinics with use of the same type of IUD is sometimes greater than the difference in event rates for different IUD types used in the same clinic. This can occur because varying client populations, provider skills, and attitudes all influence study results. Comparative IUD studies all done at the same site are therefore the most useful for evaluation but have rarely been organized on a large scale.

To provide a clearer focus in this chapter, we have limited our presentation to the most widely used IUDs—the Lippes Loop, the Saf-T-Coil, the Copper T, the Cooper 7, and the Multiload Cu250.

DEVICE DESIGN

Physiology

Before the contraceptive effect of IUD is examined, a brief review of normal reproductive physiology is helpful. The ovum is expelled from the follicle on the ovarian surface around the middle of the menstrual cycle—this is called *ovulation*. The ovum then travels down the fallopian tube, where fertilization may occur. The ovum is capable of being fertizilized for only 1 day, but the spermatozoa are capable of fertilizing for several days. Following coitus the spermatozoa find their way into the fallopian tubes through their own action and the muscular activity of the uterus (Figure 3-2).

After fertilization the egg continues its 3-day journey down to the uterine cavity. During this period the ovum undergoes several

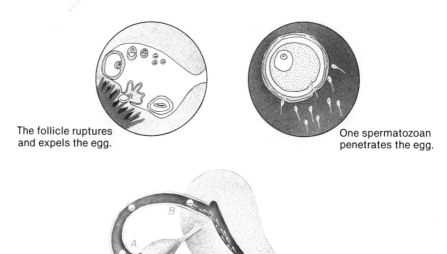

The follicle ruptures and expels the egg.

One spermatozoan penetrates the egg.

Figure 3-2. *Ovulation (A) and fertilization (B).*

stages of cell division as it becomes a *blastocyst*—a tiny fluid-filled ball of over 100 cells. The remains of the ovarian follicle form the corpus luteum, which produces hormones to support the developing blastocyst. Implantation occurs sometime after the blastocyst arrives in the uterine cavity. The exact timing of this event is not known but probably occurs between the seventh and ninth day after fertilization. Sometime during this reproductive process, the IUD exerts its contraceptive effect.

Contraceptive Mechanism

The precise reason why IUDs prevent pregnancy is unknown. Many explanations have been proposed, but there is no single hypothesis that satisfactorily explains the numerous physiological actions of IUDs that have been observed in humans. Intrauterine devices do not disturb the basic functioning of the menstrual cycle, and there is no alteration of ovulation, ovum transport, or the function of the corpus luteum in women using an IUD.

The most widely accepted explanation of the the contraceptive effect of the IUD has been that it acts as a "foreign body" in the uterus. A "foreign body" is defined as any object or material not normally found in a physiological environment. The presence of such an object within a human body stimulates an inflammatory reaction somewhat similar to an infection. In the case of the IUD, this reaction is "sterile" (*not* caused by bacteria or viruses) and is produced inside the uterine cavity, rendering the endometrial lining inhospitable for implantation of the ovum. This reaction has been documented in laboratory studies and, in the absence of proven alternatives, remains the best explanation of the IUD's contraceptive effect.

The contraceptive efficacy of the smaller copper IUDs may be due to the copper causing an even greater inflammatory response within the uterine cavity. Copper may also cause biochemical alterations in the endometrial lining by inhibiting the normal functioning of enzymes, thus preventing implantation of the ovum. In addition, copper ions released into the uterine cavity from the device may liquefy the secretions of endometrial cells, reducing the stickiness of the endometrial surface and making implantation more difficult.

Design

The design of a particular intrauterine device is an important factor in determining its contraceptive effectiveness. For a device to be successful as a contraceptive, the design must produce a low pregnancy rate and satisfactory retention of the device without troublesome side-effects. Several contradictory features must be reconciled in the design of the ideal IUD:

- It should be easy to insert but be resistant to expulsion.
- It should fit the average size uterus, but not overdistend small uteri.
- The endometrial reaction caused by the device must effectively prevent pregnancy but not be associated with complications.

As a rule, large IUDs have the lowest pregnancy and expulsion rates but are associated with a higher frequency of side-effects and thus must be removed more often. Conversely, small devices usually have higher pregnancy and expulsion rates but less frequent removals for side-effects. The addition of copper to IUDs has changed this rule and allows the use of small, flexible devices that are easily inserted and well tolerated but that at the same time retain low pregnancy and expulsion rates.

Currently available IUDs may be divided into two general categories—nonmedicated and medicated. The Lippes Loop and the
Saf-T-Coil are the most successful examples of nonmedicated devices. Medicated devices are so described because they release a
substance that alters the uterine environment, and those currently
used are copper-bearing (Copper T, Copper 7, and Multiload Cu250)
or, rarely, hormone-releasing. Because the hormone-releasing devices are more expensive and so far offer few advantages over other
devices, they are not discussed further in this chapter.

Nonmedicated. The Lippes Loop (Ortho Pharmaceutical Company, U.S.A.) is an "S"-shaped device made of flexible polyethylene
plastic (Figure 3-3). After being inserted into the uterine cavity
through a straight plastic inserter tube, it reassumes its original
shape. This device was one of the first to have a small amount of
barium added to its plastic to ensure visibility on x-ray. This is now
done for all IUDs. In addition, the Lippes Loop was the first flexible
IUD to have a string of plastic thread that extends out through the
cervix and into the vagina, allowing the user to check the presence
of the device. The string also aids in removal of the IUD and is
standard on all IUDs.

The Lippes Loop is available in four sizes, but the smaller two,
labeled "A" and "B," have undesirably high rates of pregnancy and
expulsion and are not recommended for wide use. The two most
commonly used sizes are labeled "C" and "D." The "D"-size loop,
identified by its white tail (Table 3-1), is recommended for use in
most multiparous women. It is particularly useful for long-term
contraception and is the standard device used on a worldwide basis
in family planning services. The size "C" loop, identified by its yellow tail, it recommended for women who experience excessive
bleeding and pain with the "D"-size loop.

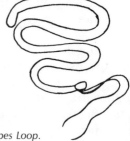

Figure 3-3. *The Lippes Loop.*

Table 3-1.
Identification of IUD Strings by Device and Color.

	Number	Color	Color	Number	
Lippes Loop C	1 or 2	Yellow	Blue-green	2	**Saf-T-Coil**
Lippes Loop D	1 or 2	White	Black	1	**Copper 7**
Saf-T-Coil	2	Blue-green	Light blue	2	**Copper T or**
					Multiload Cu250
Copper T	2	Light blue	Yellow	1 or 2	**Lippes Loop C**
Copper 7	1	Black or	White	1	**Lippes Loop D or**
		white			**Copper 7**
Multiload	2	Light blue or		2	**Lippes Loop D or**
Cu250		white			**Multiload Cu250**

The Lippes Loop D has been extensively studied by many investigators, including the Cooperative Statistical Program (CSP) of The Population Council, and a great deal of information has been accumulated. Comparative event rates for all major IUD designs are listed in Table 3-2. Cooperative Statistical Program data on the Loop D revealed a first-year continuation rate of 77%. Rates of discontinuation for all reasons were markedly reduced after the first year of loop use, as they are in users of all types of IUDs. After 6 years of use the cumulative continuation rate in Loop D users was 43%—a figure demonstrating a high degree of satisfactory long-term contraceptive use.

Recent research indicates that the Lippes Loop may not remain fully effective and free of side-effects indefinitely as once was as-

Table 3-2.
Comparative IUD Event Rates.

	Pregnancy	Expulsion	Removals for Bleeding and Pain	Continuation (%)
Lippes Loop D	2–2.5	7–10	7.5–12	75–85
Saf-T-Coil	0.5–3	7.5–19	4–14.5	70–88
Copper T	1–3	2–9.5	4.5–12	76–86
Copper 7	1.5–3	5–15	1.5–11	66–75
Multiload Cu250	0.5–4	2–2.5	3–4	81–91

Rates are net events per 100 women in first year of use.
Listed are ranges of rates from major studies.

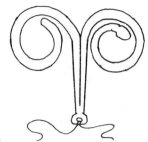

Figure 3-4. *The Saf-T-Coil.*

sumed. Loops removed after many years of use have been found to be encrusted with calcium salts, a uterine reaction that affects medicated and nonmedicated devices alike. This buildup of deposits may reduce the device's contraceptive effectiveness and/or cause the user intermenstrual bleeding or discomfort. Apparently these problems will generally occur much later with use of the loop than with that of the copper devices. Thus the effectiveness of the Lippes Loop may be finite. Providers should watch for side-effects in loop wearers possibly developing after many years of satisfactory use.

The Saf-T-Coil or "double coil" (Schmid, U.S.A.) is also made of flexible polyethylene plastic (Figure 3-4). The Saf-T-Coil is no longer manufactured, but health providers in family planning will continue to see women with these devices. As with the Lippes Loop, the Saf-T-Coil was made in different sizes to accommodate variations in uterine size. The Saf-T-Coil has two blue-green strings, regardless of size.

Studies of the Saf-T-Coil have found it to be a very serviceable device. First-year event rates determined through the CSP found a continuation rate of 69.5%. Long-range studies of the Saf-T-Coil, like those for the Lippes Loop, have shown a reduction in discontinuation over time. This device was chosen primarily by providers in the United States, where experience has been quite favorable.

Medicated. The Copper T (Searle, U.S.A.) is a polyethylene plastic T-shaped device with fine copper wire wrapped around the vertical shaft, providing a surface area from which copper ions are released into the intrauterine environment (Figure 3-5). The Copper T has two light-blue strings. Studies comparing the Copper T with a plain "T"-shaped device demonstrate markedly increased contraceptive effectiveness from the addition of copper. In one study, the first-year pregnancy rate for the plain T was 18%, whereas the Cop-

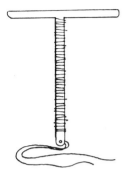

Figure 3-5. *The Copper T.*

per T had a pregnancy rate between 1% and 2%. In the United
States, clinical experience with the Copper T has found a continuation rate of 76% for the first year of use.

It has been demonstrated that increasing the amount of copper
released by an IUD increases its contraceptive effectiveness. Currently available copper intrauterine devices generally have a copper
surface area of 200–250 mm². It is recommended that they be
changed every 3–4 years because oxidation and crusting develops
on the copper wire, which creates a barrier to the dispersion of the
copper ions into the uterine cavity. This can reduce the contraceptive effectiveness of the devices to an unacceptable level. Some long-
term studies, however, have shown that both the Copper T and the
Copper 7 can continue to provide safe and effective contraception
when left in place for up to 6 years.

There does not seem to be any particular reason for preferring
the Copper T over the Lippes Loop in multiparous women, although
a 1982 World Health Organization (WHO) study recommends the
Copper T-220C over both the Lippes Loop and the Copper 7. The
Lippes Loop is less expensive than the copper IUDs and does not
have to be changed every 3 years. The D Loop would appear to be
the device of choice for most family planning services in which
arrangement for reinsertion is difficult and adds too much to service
costs.

The Copper 7 or "Gravigard" (Searle, U.S.A.) is a polypropylene
device with 200 mm² of copper surface area exposed from fine copper wire wrapped around the vertical shaft (Figure 3-6). It has one
string, either black or white. The Copper 7 is the same length as the
Copper T (36 mm) but is slightly smaller in width (28 mm compared
with 32 mm). At the meeting of the two arms of the Copper 7, there
is a small rounded cap that seals the arms together and protects

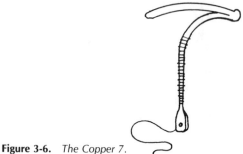

Figure 3-6.   *The Copper 7.*

against perforation of the uterus. The diameter of a folded Copper 7 is smaller than that of a Copper T, and thus the Copper 7 is easier to insert through a small cervical os.

Both the Copper 7 and the Copper T have roughly similar satisfactory event rates. Clinical studies of the Copper 7 have found a first-year continuation rate of 75%.

The Multiload Cu250 (Organon, U.K.) is being marketed in Europe, Canada, and other countries. The Multiload is another copper-releasing device with copper wire wrapped around its vertical shaft, exposing a copper surface area of 250 mm^2 (Figure 3-7). The arms of the Multiload Cu250 are extremely flexible serrated plastic fins that form a somewhat omega (Ω) shape and hold the device in place without stretching the uterine cavity. Bleedings and cramping are apparently minimized by this design, and the expulsion rate is reported to be very low. A study of 2782 insertions covering almost 30,000 woman-months of use show impressive first-year event rates: pregnancy, less than 1%; expulsion, 2%; and removals for bleeding and pain, 4%. A smaller study found a higher pregnancy rate (3.9%), but other event rates were very low. Continuation rates have been

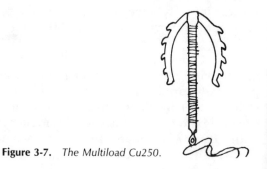

Figure 3-7.   *The Multiload Cu250.*

reported to be above 80%. Insertion of the Multiload Cu250 is very simple and does not require a plunger, thus reducing the possibility of uterine perforation. Clinical studies seem to indicate that this device will retain high contraceptive effectiveness for 4 years or more without replacement.

INSERTION PROCEDURE

An IUD can be used by most multiparous women who desire effective long-term contraception. Prior to insertion of an IUD, however, there must be thorough counseling and an adequate medical history and pelvic examination to determine whether the IUD is the best contraceptive alternative for that individual. These steps are very important to help ensure that each woman who elects to have an IUD will be a satisfied client.

Counseling Considerations

Sensitive and thorough counseling is integrally related to better client tolerance of IUD insertion and successful long-term use (see Chapter 1). The prospective IUD user should be told that the IUD is second only to the pill in contraceptive effectiveness, without the potential complications associated with hormonal contraception and without the need for remembering daily to take a medication. Use of the IUD is associated with its own set of side-effects, however, which should be explained.

Resistance to IUD use may occur for surprisingly simple reasons. Some women may be mistrustful of the devices themselves, and be hesitant to have a piece of plastic inside their bodies. Some women may simply feel uneasy about upsetting a natural process by using contraception. One aspect of IUD use often regarded as a major advantage is that it disassociates contraception from the sex act. Some women, however, may not understand how it is possible for the device to prevent conception if it is not used in direct connection with intercourse. These concerns should be fully explored during the counseling session, along with the method's advantages and disadvantages.

Risks associated with IUD use should neither be ignored nor exaggerated. Myths regarding IUDs should be brought into the open. It should be emphasized that IUDs do *not* cause cancer, nor do they cause a deformed baby if a woman becomes pregnant with an IUD in place. If such a pregnancy occurs, the IUD probably will be removed to reduce the possibility of uterine infection (see page 116). The woman should also understand that if at any time she is dissatisfied with her IUD and wants to have it removed, this will be done immediately on her request.

Once a client has decided to use an IUD, she should be counseled about the insertion procedure itself. Some women are fearful that the insertion may be painful; the woman can minimize any discomfort during the procedure by relaxing as much as possible. If the woman knows what to expect during the IUD insertion and afterward, she is less likely to be upset about possible side-effects.

Subsequent fertility. Return to normal fertility after IUD removal is rapid. Of women trying to conceive after IUD use, 75% do so within 6 months and 85%–90% within 1 year. This rate is comparable to that found in women discontinuing the use of barrier methods and is higher than that for women stopping oral contraceptives. There is no effect on the offspring of former IUD users.

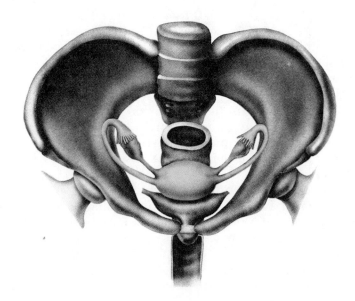

Figure 3-8. *The uterus lies in the pelvic cavity.*

Anatomy

Clinical personnel inserting IUDs must be thoroughly familiar with female reproductive anatomy. The uterus is a pear-shaped organ composed primarily of involuntary muscle called the *myometrium*. Its cavity is lined by a mucous membrane called the *endometrium*. The uterus lies in the pelvic cavity, between the urinary bladder and the rectosigmoid colon (Figure 3-8). Its precise position and contour, however, are subject to much individual variation and are dependent on genetic, pathological, and developmental factors. Uteri normally vary in characteristics of flexion, version, size, and configuration.

The uterus usually lies somewhat curved on its long axis. This is called *flexion*. When curved up toward the urinary bladder, the position of the uterus is called *anteflexion*. *Retroflexion* is the term used to describe a uterus that curves backward toward the rectosigmoid colon (Figure 3-9).

Version is another term used to describe uterine position. It describes the position of the whole uterine structure in relation to the long axis of the vagina. In most cases the uterus is found in the anteverted position, meaning that the long axis (the length) of the uterus is directed more upward than the long axis of the vagina. Retroversion is a less common, but still quite normal, position. A retroverted uterus projects backward, almost in line with the vaginal axis (Figure 3-10).

The *size* and *configuration* of the uterus are dependent mainly on the parity of the woman, although again, genetic, developmental, and pathological factors cause individual differences. In a young girl before puberty, or in the mature woman who continues to have an infantile uterus, the cervix is the dominant portion of the organ—comprising about two-thirds of the length of the uterus—with the corpus or uterine body comprising the other one-third. In the parous woman the ratio is reversed, with the corpus accounting for about two-thirds of the total uterine length. The adult nulliparous uterus lies in the intermediate range—half cervix and half corpus (see Figure 5-3). The parous uterus is also somewhat larger in its overall dimensions than the nulliparous uterus.

The appearance of the cervix is also changed with parity. In the nulliparous woman, the cervix appears essentially round to oval in shape, and the external os is distinctly round. The parous woman has a more slitlike opening at the external os with the overall shape of the cervix somewhat more flattened (see Figure 5-4). The cervix

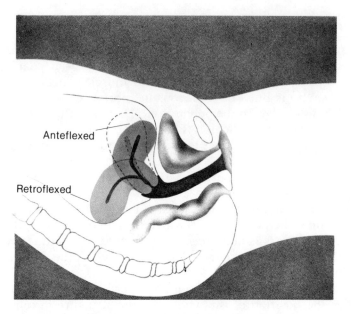

Figure 3-9. *Uterine flexion.*

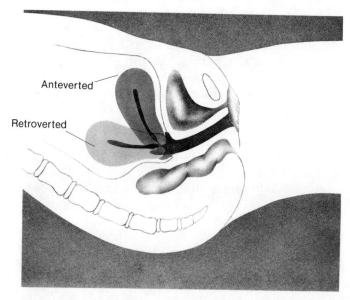

Figure 3-10. *Uterine version. An anteverted uterus is most common.*

90

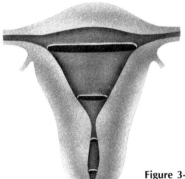

Figure 3-11. *The cervical canal is cylindrical, whereas the uterine cavity is triangular and flat.*

that has been previously dilated by childbirth is generally more elastic and is easily manipulated and dilated.

The uterine cavity is somewhat triangular in shape, with the apex of the triangle at the internal os of the cervix. The base of the triangle (the farthest wall of the uterus) is the uterine fundus, and the cavity itself is flattened from front to back (Figure 3-11).

An essential function of the preinsertion pelvic examination is to look for these variations in size and position, to ensure both that the proper device design is chosen for the individual woman and that the proper insertion technique is carefully followed.

Client Screening

History and examination. Prior to insertion of an IUD, a medical history must be taken and a bimanual pelvic examination performed to detect any possible contraindications to IUD use. It is appropriate and sometimes preferable for the history to be taken and pelvic examination performed by a nurse-midwife, family planning nurse, or other specially trained nonphysician. If any questions remain, the woman should be referred to a physician for a final decision on whether an IUD should be inserted.

Bimanual pelvic examination should determine the size, shape, and position of the uterus as well as cervical and uterine texture. With the woman on an examining table in the lithotomy position, the provider begins by separating the labia minora and depressing the perineum with two fingers of a gloved hand. The fingers are gently introduced into the vagina until the cervix is reached. The fingers of the opposite hand stabilize the pelvic contents by means

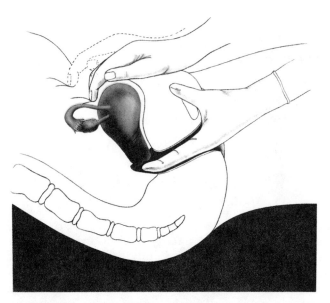

Figure 3-12. *Bimanual examination. By sweeping the hand on the abdomen toward the pubic bone, the examiner can palpate the uterine fundus and estimate its size.*

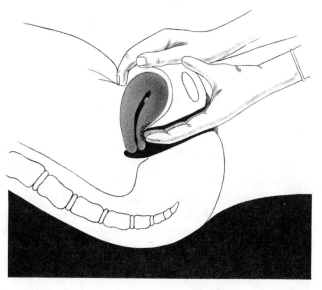

Figure 3-13. *Hegar's sign—when the uterine isthmus feels discontinuous—is an early sign of pregnancy.*

of gentle pressure through the abdominal wall. If gentle motion of the cervix or corpus causes the woman to feel tenderness or pain, there may be acute or chronic inflammation that could in some cases contraindicate IUD insertion.

With the vaginal fingers stablizing the cervix as a reference point, the uterine fundus is palpated by placing the other hand on the upper abdomen and sweeping it toward the pubic bone (Figure 3-12). A normally positioned uterus can be felt between the two hands. If the uterus is retroflexed or retroverted, it may not be palpable from the abdomen, but can be felt by gently stretching the posterior vaginal vault with the examining finger. Determination of version and flexion is important to ensure safe uterine sounding.

With the uterus positioned between the two hands, the examiner can make a fairly accurate estimation of uterine size. Since pregnancy is an absolute contraindication to IUD insertion, the examiner must check carefully for any signs of unusual uterine enlargement. In the first weeks of pregnancy the increase in overall uterine size is almost imperceptible, but the vaginal examining fingers will detect a softening of the cervix. At 6 weeks since the last normal menstrual period, this cervical softening will feel doughy, and the lower uterine corpus will also soften. Then the area between the cervix and the corpus—the isthmus—will become so soft as to make the uterus seem discontinuous and unusually flexible. This is called *Hegar's sign* and indicates a pregnancy beyond 6 weeks (Figure 3-13). If the pregnancy is unwanted, it can be terminated (see Chapter 5) and the IUD inserted immediately thereafter.

After estimation of uterine size, the bimanual examination should proceed to the adnexa (the ovaries, tubes, and uterine ligaments). By placing both fingers of the vaginal hand on one adnexal side, and pressing with the abdominal hand, the ovary on that side can usually be felt (Figure 3-14). The normal fallopian tube will not be distinguishable. Gentleness is essential because the ovaries are usually distinctly tender. *Unusual* tenderness in the ovaries or other areas of the adnexa may indicate inflammation. Palpation of an unexpected fullness or mass may indicate ectopic pregnancy (see page 117), uterine fibroids, an ovarian cyst, or pelvic malignancy. Any such finding therefore requires further investigation before proceeding with IUD insertion.

Contraindications. The most generally recognized *absolute* contraindications to IUD insertion (those conditions that present a serious health risk to the woman if she uses an IUD) are:

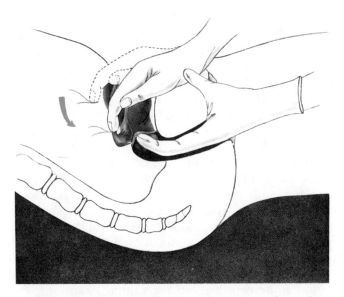

Figure 3-14. *Palpation of the tubes and ovaries must be gentle.*

- Known or suspected pregnancy.
- Known or suspected cervical or uterine malignancy (cancer). (*Note:* cervical dysplasia is *not* an absolute contraindication to IUD use.)
- Acute or chronic pelvic infection. (See also Table 3-3.)

Relative contraindications to IUD insertion (those conditions where the possible risk must be balanced with the benefits of IUD use) include:

- Nulliparity (women who have never been pregnant; IUDs should be used in nulliparous women only when other contraceptive methods are inappropriate or unavailable and avoidance of pregnancy is important to the woman's health).
- Dysmenorrhea (painful menstruation).
- Menorrhagia (heavy menstruation), metrorrhagia (irregular bleeding), or both.
- Abnormalities of uterine size, shape, or position, including a bicornuate (divided) uterus, very small uterus, or uterine fibroids (benign growths) causing enlargement or distortion of the uterus.
- History of pelvic infection.

- History of ectopic pregnancy.
- Severe cervicitis (infection of the cervix) or cervical stenosis.
- Anemia (see page 108).
- Valvular heart disease (an infection developing from IUD use could cause infection of the heart valves in these women).
- Anticoagulant therapy (IUD use could cause increased menstrual bleeding). (See also Table 3-3.)

Previous cesarean section is not a contraindication to IUD insertion, although some practitioners recommend the use of a copper device in these women because it can be more gently inserted with a "withdrawal" technique (see page 103).

Preexisting cervical dysplasia (benign abnormal cells) is *not* a contraindication to IUD use, and it should be emphasized again that use of an IUD does not cause cervical dysplasia or cancer, nor will it accelerate the progression of dysplasia to carcinoma in situ. If found, dysplasia can be treated with an IUD in place.

If a woman has an absolute contraindication to IUD use, a device should definitely not be inserted. For those women with relative contraindications, the potential benefits and hazards of an IUD must be carefully evaluated and an individual decision made.

Risks from contraceptive methods must always be compared to the average risks of maternal mortality and morbidity in the local context. The recent findings of increasing health risks from oral contraceptives among older women and those who smoke cigarettes (see Chapter 2) may make the IUD a desirable contraceptive method, among other alternatives. Those women who should *not* use an IUD

Table 3-3. Contraindications to IUD Insertion.	
Absolute:	
Pregnancy	
Cervical or uterine cancer	
Acute or chronic pelvic infection	
Relative:	
Nulliparity	Severe cervicitis
Dysmenorrhea	Cervical stenosis
Heavy or irregular menstruation	Anemia
Uterine abnormalities	Valvular heart disease
History of ectopic pregnancy	Anticoagulant therapy
History of pelvic infection	

must be offered another form of contraception that is appropriate for them.

Time of insertion.   An IUD may be inserted at any time during the menstrual cycle, but insertion during menstruation is preferable for several reasons:

- The likelihood of the woman being pregnant is small.
- The cervix is softer and slightly open.
- Bleeding and cramps from an IUD insertion are less noticeable during menstruation and thus are less apt to create anxiety.

It is often difficult, however, for a woman to see her health provider for an IUD insertion precisely at the time of her menstrual period, or there may even be cultural restraints on pelvic examination during the menstrual flow. In these situations, an IUD should be inserted whenever the woman is seen for examination. Otherwise she may not return for insertion later and could remain at risk of unwanted pregnancy.

Intrauterine devices may also be inserted in the postpartum period, within the first few days after delivery. The International Postpartum Program (IPP), begun by The Population Council in 1966, studied a large number of postpartum insertions. Insertion within the first week postpartum does not increase pain or infection but is associated with a relatively high expulsion rate—25% when the IUD is inserted on day of delivery, declining to 10% at 1 week. After 1 week postpartum, however, the risk of uterine perforation increases. Intrauterine device insertion should then be delayed until the postpartum visit, usually scheduled for 6 weeks after delivery. Considering these factors, the optimal time for early postpartum IUD insertion appears to be day 4 after delivery.

Researchers are attempting to perfect an IUD design that would permit insertion immediately after delivery of the placenta. One design, called the "Delta Loop," is a standard Lippes Loop with catgut knots added to the top transverse arm. The ends of these knots help anchor the device in the large postpartum uterus and then dissolve as the uterus involutes (shrinks). Studies have found that the catgut dissolves too quickly, and now the possibility is being considered of using projections of biodegradable plastic to serve the same function. These devices are inserted by hand, and the procedure must be conducted under the strictest aseptic hospital conditions. Further study is necessary before such a device is appropriate for wide use.

The IPP found that many women prefer early postpartum IUD insertions because after delivery their motivation to use family planning is great. These insertions are especially useful if women are not as likely to return for a postpartum visit and may lose contact altogether with a family planning service.

The postpartum visit to the hospital, clinic, or practitioner is another ideal time for IUD insertion. The woman is still highly motivated to accept contraception, and her uterus has returned to normal size, reducing the risk of uterine perforation. The device should be inserted before she resumes regular intercourse and becomes exposed to the risk of unwanted pregnancy.

Insertion of an IUD at the postpartum visit may be especially appropriate for women who are breastfeeding. Although lactation significantly reduces the chance of pregnancy, it is by no means a guaranteed contraceptive method. The use of combined oral contraceptives is not recommended for lactating women; an IUD can provide the breastfeeding mother with effective contraception that will continue after lactation is completed, without her needing to return to the clinic.

An IUD can also be easily inserted in conjunction with first-trimester spontaneous or therapeutic abortion. Several studies have demonstrated the efficacy of postabortal IUD insertion and have concluded that there is no difference between event rates for immediate postabortal and later postmenstrual insertion. There are no serious complications in the first month following immediate postabortal IUD insertion, although menstruation may resume earlier and be slightly heavier for these women. It should be emphasized that women with IUDs inserted immediately after uterine evacuation do *not* have a higher risk of endometritis (uterine infection) when compared to those having postmenstrual insertions. The need for effective postabortal contraception is clear when one considers that an estimated three-fourths of women will ovulate within 6 weeks after abortion.

Immediate postcoital insertion of IUDs can be used to prevent pregnancy following unprotected intercourse in the middle of the menstrual cycle. Since the fertilized ovum remains in the fallopian tube for several days, insertion of an IUD immediately after intercourse can prevent implantation of the ovum in the uterus. This method has been used in several studies employing the Copper T, Copper 7, and Multiload Cu250 devices with high degrees of effectiveness and safety. An important advantage of this method of postcoital contraception is that it is apparently effective up to 5 days after unprotected intercourse, whereas oral contraceptives must be initiated much sooner. In addition, the IUD can be left in place to provide the woman with satisfactory long-term contraception. When considering using IUDs in this manner, the health provider must, of course, screen the client for the contraindications to IUD use.

Equipment and Laboratory Tests

A simple set of basic medical equipment is necessary for IUD insertion. The quantities of each instrument required will vary according to the number of IUDs to be inserted per day at the clinic. In addition to an examining table and appropriate light source, it is desirable to have the equipment listed in Table 3-4.

Sterilization of instruments. Intrauterine device insertion requires the capability to wash and sterilize instruments. If an autoclave is not available, metal instruments can be boiled, or cold disinfection of equipment can be accomplished by soaking either in a solution of benzalkonium chloride (1:750) or an iodine solution (1:2500). Some IUDs are made available prepackaged in sterile wrappers, whereas others are supplied in bulk without prior sterilization. If necessary, the IUDs and inserters may be sterilized in a benzalkonium or iodine solution. Complete cold *sterilization* of instruments requires soaking for 5 hours in a formaldehyde or alkaline glutaraldehyde (Cidex or Sporicidin) solution. This technique requires sterile water, which may be difficult to obtain in some developing areas.

Laboratory tests. Laboratory requirements for IUD insertion are minimal. The only necessary test is a hemoglobin or hematocrit to determine the extent to which the woman may be anemic. If hemoglobin is less than 10 g/100 ml or hematocrit less than 30%, it is probably best not to insert an IUD. Since the presence of an IUD

Table 3-4. IUD Insertion Kit.
• Speculums—small, medium, and large • Tenaculum • Sponge forceps • Straight artery forceps • Uterine sound • Scissors • Surgical gloves

within the uterine cavity will usually increase menstrual flow, this may aggravate preexisting anemia. The final decision on whether to insert an IUD in an anemic woman should depend on what is considered to be significant anemia within the local medical context and on what other contraceptive methods are available to her. If the woman is anemic, appropriate treatment should of course be provided.

Intrauterine device insertions provide the opportunity for other medical tests. If facilities are available to perform and evaluate Papanicolaou smears, one should be done prior to IUD insertion for purposes of cancer screening. A Pap smear is only a desirable adjunct, however, and is by no means a prerequisite for IUD insertion. Sexually transmitted diseases, especially gonorrhea, are a much greater problem than cancer for young women, and if at all possible, a culture for gonorrhea should be taken at IUD insertion. If the test is positive for gonoccocal organisms, immediate treatment with penicillin or other appropriate antibiotics should be given to combat this potentially serious disease (see Chapter 7). Early elimination of the gonorrhea will also reduce the possibility of the IUD aggravating a preexisting infection.

Insertion Technique

The techniques for IUD insertion vary according to the specific device being used, and the peculiarities of each design's technique are discussed later. The following applies to insertion of *all* IUDs.

Sounding. With the vaginal speculum in place, the cervix is cleansed with an antiseptic solution such as benzalkonium chloride or iodine. The cervix is grasped with a single tooth tenaculum, and gentle traction is applied to straighten the axis of the uterus. Then the uterus is gently sounded to determine the *depth* and *direction* of the uterine cavity (Figure 3-15). This will ensure proper placement of the device without perforation or discomfort.

A malleable metal sound gives the provider the advantage of an instrument that can be shaped to match the extent and direction of flexion and version determined during the bimanual examination. Disposable plastic sounds are available but are not malleable. The sound and all other instruments that will enter the uterus must be sterile.

Some IUD inserters have a movable stop that can be set to the uterine depth found during sounding to reduce the possibility of perforation when the device is inserted. It will be unlikely to find a

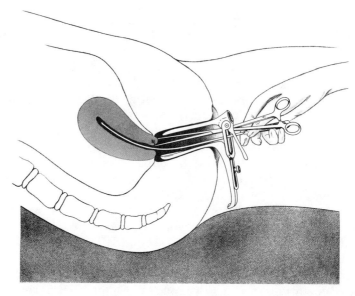

Figure 3-15. *Sounding determines the depth and direction of the uterine cavity.*

parous uterus that sounds to a depth less than 6 cm, but if this occurs, it is best not to insert an IUD, and another contraceptive method should be recommended.

Paracervical block. Occasionally, the cervical canal is very tight and must be opened with a small dilator. If dilation causes significant discomfort, a paracervical block with 5 ml of local anesthesia such as lidocaine hydrochloride 1% can be used, but it is seldom necessary. The block is injected into the upper vaginal wall next to the cervix at the 4 o'clock and 8 o'clock positions at an approximate depth of 0.5 cm beneath the vaginal surface (see Figure 5-16).

Insertion. The IUD is loaded into the inserter under sterile conditions. It is important to insert the IUD immediately after it has been loaded into the inserter; otherwise, the plastic will lose its "memory" and the device will not return to its original shape. With gentle traction on the tenaculum, the inserter is placed through the cervical canal and into the uterine cavity. Insertion of the IUD is then accomplished according to the specifc instructions for the device design, making sure that the device is placed high in the uterine fundus. The IUD string is cut so that approximately 2.5 cm (1 in.)

Table 3-5. IUD Insertion Diameters.	
	Diameter of Inserter (mm)
Copper 7	3.1
Multiload Cu250	3.5
Saf-T-Coil (small)	3.8
Saf-T-Coil (large)	4.5
Lippes Loop (all sizes)	5.3
Copper T	6.0

protrudes through the external cervical os. The insertion procedure has now been completed, and all instruments are removed from the vagina.

Generally, the narrower the diameter of the inserter, the easier and less traumatic the insertion process will be. The width of the inserter of course depends on the size and design of the IUD being used. If it is necessary to insert an IUD in a nulliparous woman, the small flexible Copper 7 or the smallest Saf-T-Coil would appear to be the easiest and least traumatic to insert through a nulliparous cervix, since their insertion diameters are much smaller than those of other devices (Table 3-5).

Push-in for loop and coil. There are two basic techniques for IUD insertion: a *push-in* technique and a *withdrawal* technique. The push-in technique is used for the Lippes Loop and Saf-T-Coil. After the device is loaded so that it will open into the plane of the uterine cavity (Figure 3-16), the inserter is passed through the cervix and placed high in the uterine cavity. The plunger is pushed, releasing

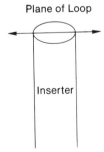

Plane of Loop

Inserter

Figure 3-16. *The plane of the loop must match the uterine plane.*

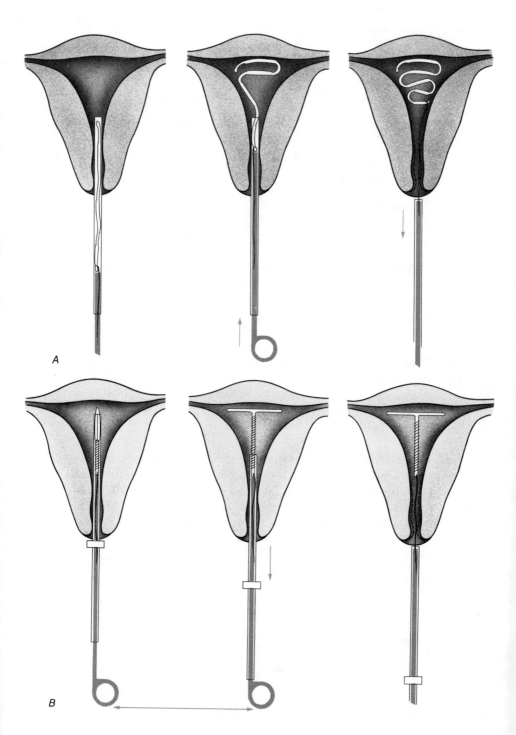

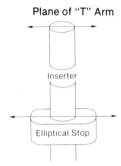

Plane of "T" Arm

Inserter

Elliptical Stop

Figure 3-18. *The plane of the "T" arm must match the plane of the inserter's stop.*

the IUD from the inserter. The plunger and inserter are then re-moved together (Figure 3-17A).

Withdrawal for Copper T and 7. The withdrawal technique is used for the Copper 7 and Copper T devices. When the T or the 7 is loaded, the elliptical stop on the inserter (previously set to the sounding depth) should be adjusted to match the plane of the de-vice's transverse arms (Figure 3-18). Using the stop as a guide, the provider will be able to ensure that the device opens up in the uterine plane.

The inserter is placed in the uterine cavity and gently advanced until the top of the fundus is felt. Then the inserter is withdrawn while the plunger holds the IUD in place (Figure 3-17B). The with-drawal technique reduces the chance of uterus perforation and en-sures *high fundal placement,* which should be the goal when inserting any IUD (Table 3-6). High fundal placement enhances contraceptive effectiveness and reduces the likelihood of expulsion.

The Multiload Cu250 has an inserter, but no plunger. The in-serter is advanced to the top of the uterine fundus and then is sim-ply withdrawn, leaving the device in place. This technique provides excellent safety and is easy to use.

Reactions to insertion. Some women who have an IUD inserted may experience transient syncope (faintness) and/or abdominal dis-comfort with cramping. The client should be advised to remain in a reclining position and usually will feel well within a few minutes. If

Figure 3-17. *(A) Push-in technique: the plunger is pushed, releasing the IUD, and the inserter is then withdrawn. (B) Withdrawal technique: the inserter is advanced to the fundus and then withdrawn, while the plunger keeps the IUD in place.*

Table 3-6. IUD Insertion: Points to Remember.
• Perform bimanual examination • Stabilize cervix with tenaculum • Sound uterus for depth and direction • Assess need for cervical dilation • Insert using proper technique—push-in or withdrawal • Ensure high fundal placement

she continues to feel faint, spirits of ammonia may be held under her nose to revive her. Atropine sulfate should be available to treat the rare but potentially serious extreme vasovagal reaction.

If the woman is bothered by abdominal cramping, mild analgesic medication such as aspirin or a prostaglandin inhibitor (see page 109) may be administered. In order to reduce such symptoms, IUD insertion must be performed in the gentlest manner possible. Sharp pain and cramping, particularly accompanied by uterine bleeding or disappearance of the IUD string, may be signs of uterine perforation (see page 111).

Follow-Up

Successful use of IUDs will be directly affected by the attitudes and practices of clinic personnel and by the quality of client care that is provided. The importance of sensitive person-to-person interactions between clients and clinic staff has been documented in studies that have revealed considerable variation in event rates between clinics using the same device. Many researchers have found that these subjective factors often have more impact on the true effectiveness of an IUD than does its design. Whenever clinic personnel are positive in their attitudes toward IUDs, have established good client rapport, and provide supportive follow-up care, IUD continuation rates and client satisfaction are generally very high.

Some increase in bleeding and cramping is normal after IUD insertion. The properly counseled client will be able to anticipate these effects and therefore probably will not be alarmed should they occur. The provider may need to give further explanations and reassurance to allay the client fears. Unusual discomfort or irregular bleeding may have clinical significance and lead to removal of the device.

Providers who place emphasis only on the number of IUD insertions achieved are not delivering good health care. Client dissatis-

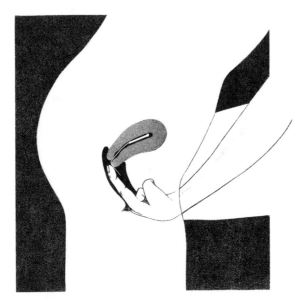

Figure 3-19. *The woman should check the IUD string after every menstruation and cramping episode and at midcycle.*

faction and device removal rates will be high. This is a special hazard for mobile family planning units, which may enthusiastically insert IUDs and then move on to other locations without returning—in effect abandoning the acceptors. A family planning service providing IUDs must deliver adequate ongoing care, which means having appropriately trained personnel for routine follow-up examinations and the facilities to deal with medical problems that might arise.

Good follow-up care begins immediately after insertion. An important part of client education is teaching the woman how to check her IUD string to verify that the device is still in place (Figure 3-19). After insertion of the device, the portion of the string that has been cut away should not be discarded, but rather given to the woman so she will know what the string feels like. To check for the string, the woman should wash her hands and reach into the vagina until the cervix is felt and the string located.

Since most IUD expulsions occur at menstruation, the woman should check for the string after each menstrual period. In addition, it is desirable for her to check for the string each month before the fertile middle period of her menstrual cycle, and also after any episode of lower abdominal cramping. If the string cannot be felt, the

---

Table 3-7.
IUD Follow-Up: Client Instructions.

1. Some increase in bleeding and cramping is normal.
2. Check for string at midcycle and after period or cramping episode.
3. If string is missing, use another contraceptive and contact health provider.
4. Also contact health provider if you have:
   • Pelvic pain or painful intercourse
   • Unusual bleeding or vaginal discharge
   • Missed a period or other sign of pregnancy
   • Chills or fever over 100.4°F
5. Return for scheduled follow-up examinations and remember time limit on medicated devices.

---

woman should refrain from intercourse or use another contraceptive method until the IUD has been checked at the family planning clinic. Having the woman check for her IUD is desirable but not mandatory and should not be aggressively urged if there are cultural objections.

Providing IUD clients with a *device identification card* is an excellent means of ensuring accurate information for follow-up care. A small, durable card should include the following information: type of device; manufacturer's lot number; date of insertion; provider's name, address, and telephone number (if applicable); source of emergency care; warning signs; and reinsertion date (if applicable). This card will remind the client of symptoms to watch for and where to go for help. The card also enables any provider to know the configuration of the device, whether it is medicated, and how long it has been in place. Warning signs for the client should include: pelvic pain or dyspareunia (painful intercourse), unusual bleeding or vaginal discharge, missed period or other sign of pregnancy, chills or fever (100.4°F or more), and a missing IUD string (Table 3-7).

The initial follow-up at the family planning clinic or other site should be performed 1–2 months following insertion. After that, the woman does not need to be seen again for a year unless she experiences interim difficulties. The woman should clearly understand that she is free to return at any time if she has any questions or problems relating to her IUD or her general health.

IUD Removal

Whenever an IUD user decides that she wishes to resume childbearing, the device is simply removed by the practitioner. Return to normal fertility after IUD removal is rapid. Removal may be necessary if the woman develops certain side-effects or complications. Removal is also recommended in menopausal women, so that irregular bleeding due to gynecological disorders will not be mistakenly ascribed to the IUD.

Removal of an IUD is usually an uncomplicated procedure. Bimanual pelvic examination should be performed to rule out pregnancy or uterine pathology. The vaginal speculum is inserted and gonoccocal culture and Pap smear obtained if indicated. The string of the IUD is visualized and grasped with uterine dressing forceps or similar instrument. Steady traction is then applied, pulling the IUD through the cervix and into the vagina. The client may experience transient discomfort and a small amount of bleeding.

If the IUD string breaks, the device may be removed from the uterine cavity with the assistance of a small hooked instrument. Flexible plastic instruments or suction cannulas can be used by trained practitioners (see Figure 5-20). Gentle probing is undertaken until the IUD is located, hooked, and removed. Occasionally, a laminaria tent may help to dilate a particularly narrow cervix prior to IUD removal. Rarely, dilation and curettage (D&C) may be necessary for removal of an embedded device.

Side-Effects

Events that may occur following IUD insertion can be categorized either as *side-effects* (Table 3-8)—normally anticipated events associated with IUD use without serious danger to the woman's health—or *complications* (Table 3-9)—abnormal events that are not generally anticipated and that may threaten the woman's health.

Bleeding. The most common side-effects of IUDs are bleeding and pain, and these are the most frequently cited medical reasons for device removal. Complaints of bleeding and pain vary according to characteristics of both the IUD and the user. In general, the greater the surface area and size of an IUD, the higher the incidence of removals for bleeding and pain. Complaints of these conditions occur most frequently among those women of low parity who would be expected to have relatively small uteri in relation to their IUD. Choosing an appropriately sized IUD can thus reduce the incidence of side-effects. Unusually heavy bleeding can also be caused by an IUD not placed high in the uterine fundus. If the device appears to be situated too low in the uterine cavity, removal and proper reinsertion may correct the bleeding problem.

Most women who have an IUD inserted will experience some changes in their menstrual flow. In general, menstruation in IUD

Table 3-8.
Side-Effects of IUD Use.
• Bleeding: heavier and/or irregular • Pain: uterine cramping

users tends to occur several days earlier, last longer, and be heavier than normal flow. Intermenstrual spotting may also occur. The mechanism for increased bleeding among IUD users is not fully understood but is probably related to several factors such as erosion of endometrial blood vessels in contact with the IUD or alteration of blood clotting mechanisms.

Bleeding patterns associated with IUD use depend somewhat on the device used. The volume of normal menstrual flow is approximately 35 ml of blood; this volume is increased in all IUD users. When a nonmedicated device is used the blood loss is about 70–80 ml. The Oxford Blood Loss Study has shown the amount of excess bleeding is less (50–60 ml) with the smaller and more flexible copper devices, which cause less distortion of the uterine cavity. The *duration* of bleeding is often longer with these copper devices, however.

Menstrual blood loss can be reduced by drugs called *prostaglandin inhibitors.* Although their primary gynecological indication has been for the treatment of dysmenorrhea, it has been shown that naproxen (Naprosyn) and ibuprofen (Motrin) can significantly reduce IUD-associated menstrual blood loss without short-term side-effects when administered during menstruation.

Some women can become anemic from increased menstrual bleeding if it is extremely heavy, or a preexisting chronic anemia can be made worse. Iron supplementation for these IUD users may be desirable.

Removals for bleeding and pain are strongly influenced by many variables, including age, parity, time of insertion, and clinic factors. The importance of clinic attitudes and practices has been discussed previously.

Cultural factors can also be important; in some societies, for instance, the occurrence of vaginal bleeding requires that a woman abstain not only from sexual activity but also from other daily routines such as food preparation or even harvesting. If the IUD is causing her prolonged menstruation or intermenstrual spotting, the social inconvenience may be a much greater problem for the woman than the physical discomfort.

Some bleeding problems associated with IUDs can be anticipated and avoided. For example, women with a history of very heavy menstruation are not good prospects for IUD use. If an IUD is nonetheless the only available method of contraception which is acceptable to the client, a copper IUD would be the device of choice. If a woman experiences unexpectedly heavy bleeding with a non-medicated device in place, switching to a copper IUD may be beneficial. The use of oral contraceptives to reduce bleeding from an IUD is *not* desirable and may only complicate evaluation of the bleeding.

For most IUD acceptors, bleeding can be handled through education, reassurance, and use of iron supplementation when necessary. If bleeding is very heavy or disrupting to the woman, however, or if she becomes anemic in spite of iron therapy, it is unwise to continue further with the IUD. It should be removed without delay and the client should be offered another contraceptive method.

Pain. The most frequent type of pain experienced by IUD users is discomfort from uterine cramping. This is caused by distention of the uterine cavity by the IUD and resultant cramping as the uterus tries to rid itself of the foreign body. Any woman who is considering IUD use must be forewarned that cramps and discomfort may occur so that she will not be surprised by these symptoms. The cramping is usually worst within the first few minutes after IUD insertion, but then subsides rapidly. There may also be increased cramping at the time of menstruation.

Severe cramps can be anticipated if the woman complains of extreme discomfort when the uterine cavity is sounded prior to IUD insertion. In these instances it may be best to recommend an alternate method of contraception if one is available. Sometimes, cramping following IUD insertion is of sufficient magnitude to necessitate immediate removal of the device.

Cramps can be minimized by gentle insertion and selection of an IUD of appropriate size that will not overdistend or place pressure on the uterine cavity. Clients who are experiencing significant discomfort with a large nonmedicated device may also benefit from switching to a smaller nonmedicated or copper IUD.

For most women, simple analgesics that inhibit the formation of prostaglandins will suffice to control cramps and other discomfort from an IUD. Common aspirin is a safe and effective prostaglandin inhibitor, as are ibuprofen (Motrin), mefenamic acid (Ponstel), naproxen (Naprosyn), naproxen sodium (Anaprox), and zomepiric sodium (Zomax). If this treatment fails, it is best to switch to another IUD or offer the woman another method of contraception rather than maintain her on powerful analgesics.

Complications

Complications of IUD use include expulsion, uterine perforation, pregnancy, ectopic pregnancy, and pelvic infection. These complications rarely occur; pregnancy or infection occurs in less than 3% of IUD users, expulsion in less than 9%, perforation in less than 1%, and ectopic pregnancy in less than 1 per 1000 users per year (Table 3-9). Nevertheless, health practitioners providing IUDs to their clients must be familiar with the symptoms of these complications and know how to manage them.

Expulsion. Expulsion is the most frequent complication of IUD use and, if undetected, places the woman at risk of pregnancy. Expulsion of the IUD results from uterine cramping and propulsion of the foreign body from the uterine cavity. Expulsions can be partial, with the IUD remaining in the lower uterine cavity or cervical canal, or the device can be completely expelled. If the firm plastic tip of the IUD is palpated at the cervical os, or if the IUD's string appears to be longer than previously noted, incomplete expulsion can be assumed. Incomplete expulsion greatly reduces contraceptive effectiveness. It may also increase the risk of uterine infection caused by bacteria ascending from the vagina if the IUD is lying in the cervical canal.

Expulsion occurs most often during the first several months of IUD use and is most common among young, low-parity women. The expulsion rate declines with increasing age and parity and duration of IUD use. In general, the smaller the device, the higher will be the rate of expulsion. For example, studies with the Lippes Loop over 1 year of use have shown 19 expulsions per 100 woman-years of use for the thinner Loop C, in comparison to 9.5 expulsions per 100 woman-years for the thicker Loop D. The addition of copper to IUDs allows for the use of smaller, better tolerated devices without increased expulsion rates. Comparative studies between the Lippes Loop and the smaller Copper T have shown essentially similar expulsion rates despite their differences in size (see Table 3-2).

The occurrence of IUD expulsion is related in part to the degree of skill of the person inserting the device and can be minimized by careful high fundal placement. The timing of insertion is also important, with higher rates of expulsion sometimes experienced if an IUD is inserted right after delivery or abortion. Despite higher postpartum and postabortal expulsion rates, insertion at this time can still provide substantial benefit. Furthermore, clinical experience

Table 3-9. Complications of IUD Use.	
	Incidence*
• Expulsion	2–10
• Perforation	1
• Intrauterine pregnancy	1–3
• Ectopic pregnancy	0.1
• Pelvic infection	3
Incidence per 100 woman-years of use.	

has shown that women in the postpartum period are highly motivated to return for reinsertion if their first device is expelled.

Expulsions are not a serious problem *if* they are detected, but unfortunately, approximately 20% of expulsions are not. Rare as pregnancy failures are with the IUD, it is estimated that one-third of the failures will occur after an unnoticed expulsion. This is why it is important to teach each woman to check for her IUD string. If no string is felt, there is the possibility of complete expulsion; if firm plastic is felt at the cervix, the woman may have a partial expulsion. In either event, the woman should return to the clinic as soon as possible and refrain from intercourse or use another method of contraception in the meantime.

Women who have expelled an IUD can have another device inserted. If the expelled IUD was small, a larger device may be beneficial. For reasons not clearly understood, many women who have a reinsertion after IUD expulsion do not again expel the device.

Perforation.   Uterine perforation is a potentially serious complication of IUD insertion. The true incidence of perforation is difficult to determine because most women with perforations are asymptomatic and the condition remains undetected. In the Cooperative Statistical Program, perforation was estimated at less than 1.2 times per 1000 insertions. Other estimates range up to 8 perforations per 1000 insertions.

The degree of the risk of perforation varies with size, shape, and consistency of the device; technique of insertion; status and configuration of the uterus; and the skill, dexterity, and experience of the practitioner. Of all these factors, the last is probably the most important. Perforations can best be avoided by meticulous IUD inser-

Table 3-10.
Management of a Missing IUD String.

The string of the IUD protruding into the vagina may be found to be missing either by the woman through self-examination or by the practitioner at a follow-up examination. A missing string can mean several things. Usually the device is still in utero, and the properly trained provider can find it and retrieve it. Occasionally a missing string may indicate expulsion, perforation, or sometimes even pregnancy. Management of a missing string should include the following steps:

1. Careful **pelvic examination** should be performed to rule out pregnancy. A urine pregnancy test may also be helpful. If the woman is pregnant she will need special management (see page 115).

2. If the woman is not pregnant, gently **probe the cervical canal** in an attempt to locate the missing string. A cotton swab is particularly suited to this purpose—not only to remove secretions, but also for catching a missing string by twirling the swab in the cervical canal. If the IUD string is located and found to be too short, the device may be removed and a new one with a longer string can be inserted.

3. If the string or device is not found in the cervix, gently **probe the uterine cavity** with a uterine sound or dressing forceps. If present, the IUD will usually be felt as a firm, grating sensation that is different from the soft, velvety feeling of the endometrium. Several flexible, corkscrewlike, plastic instruments, such as the Mi-Mark Helix, have been used to retrieve IUDs with missing strings as atraumatically as possible. The Karman uterine aspiration cannula without its syringe (see Chapter 5) can also be used by personnel familiar with this instrument to hook the IUD and remove it.

tion, and especially through careful sounding of the uterus and use of a tenaculum to straighten the uterine axis. This will ensure that the IUD is properly inserted in the uterine plane (see page 99).

Perforation rates vary depending on the insertion technique used, occurring more often when the push-in method is used with the nonmedicated devices. Perforation is less frequent with the withdrawal insertion technique used for copper devices, but this may be related in part to the fact that copper devices are simply smaller and more flexible.

Perforations occur more frequently in retroverted or retroflexed uteri. They are also more frequent when the uterine cavity has abnormal contours that are not anticipated. Some researchers note there may be a higher risk of perforation following cesarean section, when there may be thinning or scarring of the uterine wall, and they recommend using those devices that require the withdrawal technique for insertion in these women. Perforations may occur more

4. **X-ray methods** can be used to locate the IUD if it has not been expelled. The following procedures may be helpful but are more elaborate and may not be available in some facilities. Radiation of the ovaries should always be minimized in these procedures:

   a. **Abdominal x-ray.** If the IUD is not present on x-ray, expulsion can be assumed, and no further studies are necessary. If the IUD is seen on this film, additional evaluation may be necessary to determine its location as follows:

   b. **Double IUD procedure.** A device of different design is inserted into the uterine cavity and anteroposterior and lateral x-rays are taken. If the sought-after IUD is present but is not lying in the same plane as the second device just inserted it can be assumed that there has been a uterine perforation.

   c. **Uterine sound procedure.** This is similar to step b except that a uterine sound is inserted into the uterus and the x-rays are taken to determine IUD location.

   d. **Hysterosalpingogram.** This procedure requires injection of a dye into the uterine cavity and will reveal location of the IUD on x-ray.

5. **Ultrasound,** if available, can sometimes by used by specially trained personnel to help locate missing IUDs, but it is not always reliable.

If the IUD is determined to be in place within the uterine cavity, it is best to remove it and reinsert another device that will have a visible and palpable string. Removal can usually be performed with uterine dressing forceps or hooked instruments. Laminaria tents are useful for dilation of the cervix if IUD removal is difficult, but on occasion it may be necessary to perform dilation and curettage (D&C) for removal of an embedded device.

---

frequently if IUDs are inserted in the immediate postpartum or post-abortal period, but this again depends on the practitioner's skill. The possible increased risk must be weighed with the contraceptive benefits.

Uterine perforations may be either fundal or cervical, with the fundal perforations having the greater clinical significance. *Fundal* perforation results from the IUD being inserted in such a manner that it penetrates through the myometrium (uterine muscle) and out into the abdominal cavity. Delayed perforation may also occur when a device that has been inserted into the myometrium is then slowly pushed through the uterine wall by uterine contractions.

It is often difficult to determine whether a uterine perforation has occurred. A missing IUD string may be one clue but is not conclusive evidence (Table 3-10). A history of sharp, severe pain can be suggestive of, but certainly not diagnostic of, uterine perforation. Other symptoms or conditions that raise the possibility of uterine perforation by an IUD are abnormal bleeding, persistent cramping, bowel obstruction, pelvic infection, or pregnancy.

Once an IUD is determined to have perforated the uterus, there is some controversy as to whether it should be removed or left in place. Nonmedicated devices do not automatically require surgical removal. Indeed, serious complications have occurred following unwise attempts at removing these devices; they should not be removed unless the woman is very anxious or is experiencing symptoms from the perforation. Naturally, if a device that has perforated is left in place, the woman must use another form of contraception if she still wishes to avoid pregnancy. If a decision is made to remove a nonmedicated device, this can often be accomplished by laparoscopy (through a small abdominal incision), although laparatomy (major abdominal surgery) may be necessary.

Copper intrauterine devices are best removed because the metal evokes considerable tissue reaction in the abdominal cavity with subsequent formation of adhesions. Laparotomy is the method of choice for removal of these devices.

Cervical perforations can also occur with any of the IUDs discussed here. The tip of the device may push downward and, with uterine contractions, gradually become lodged in the body of the cervix. Cervical perforations are usually asymptomatic.

If a cervical perforation occurs, the IUD must be grasped and pushed upward into the uterine cavity to free the tip, and then it can be removed downward in a routine manner. Experience with this type of problem has led to modification of the Copper T device by addition of a rounded plastic ball to its lower tip in order to reduce the possibility of cervical perforation.

Intrauterine pregnancy.   Intrauterine devices provide excellent contraceptive protection but are not 100% effective. A pregnancy will occur in approximately 1%–3% of IUD users (see Table 3-2). The contraceptive failure of an IUD can lead to psychological and physical distress regardless of whether the woman wants to remain pregnant. Pregnancy may occur after uterine perforation or undetected expulsion—events that negate the contraceptive effectiveness of the device. No special hazards will be posed for the resultant pregnancy in these instances since the IUD is no longer present in the uterine cavity. More often when a woman becomes pregnant with an IUD, the device is still in place within the uterus. This is potentially far more serious since it exposes the woman to increased risk of spontaneous abortion and intrauterine sepsis (infection).

Pregnancy rates in IUD users are highest for younger women and decline with increasing age. This is probably a reflection of the biological fact that young women are generally more fertile than older ones. Likewise, among women of the same age, those of higher parity (greater demonstrated fertility) will have a greater likelihood of a pregnancy with an IUD in place. Pregnancy rates among IUD users also vary according to the degree of skill of the person inserting the device. High fundal placement is particularly important so that the device does not move downward in the uterus, leading to significant reduction in contraceptive effectiveness.

Women sometimes express fear about the possibility of a deformed baby if conception should occur with an IUD in place. No studies have found an effect with either nonmedicated or copper devices. Although pregnancy with an IUD in situ is a serious condition, women should be reassured that there is no evidence suggesting that congenital deformities are one of the resultant hazards.

If pregnancy does occur with the IUD in place, both practitioner and client are confronted with a number of important decisions—decisions that should be made early in the first trimester (Figure 3-20). Since the occurrence of pregnancy in an IUD user is by definition unplanned, many women will not desire to complete this pregnancy. Therapeutic abortion and IUD removal should be performed without delay if it is legally acceptable and desired by the woman.

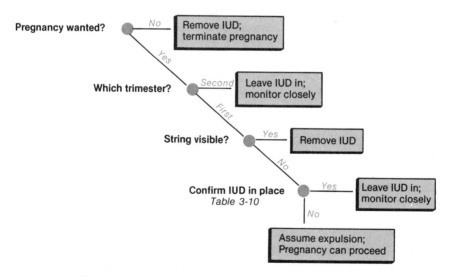

Figure 3-20. *Management of pregnancy with an IUD in place.*

If the woman wants to continue with the pregnancy, the next factor to be considered is gestational age. If she is in her second trimester of pregnancy, the IUD should *not* be removed because of the significantly increased risk of spontaneous abortion following removal at that advanced gestation. The woman must be monitored closely throughout the remainder of her pregnancy.

If the woman is in the first trimester, the provider must then check to see if the IUD string is visible. If it is visible, the device should be removed immediately. These women will have the best prognosis for completing a pregnancy started with an IUD in situ.

If the string is *not* visible, the provider must seek to confirm that the IUD is still in place. With no visible string, the practitioner cannot know if the device is embedded or has perforated the uterus. Blind manipulation of instruments in the uterus and misguided efforts to remove the IUD may only result in incomplete induced abortion, with accompanying bleeding and risk of sepsis. Confirmation of IUD placement may require referral to a facility with the proper diagnostic tools (see Table 3-10). If it is found that the IUD was previously expelled, the pregnancy can continue normally, but if the IUD *is* found in situ, it should *not* be removed. Again, the provider will need to monitor the pregnancy closely.

A woman who wants to proceed with a pregnancy with an IUD in situ should be fully informed of the attendant risks. Therapeutic abortion must be offered, after which she could pursue a normal pregnancy without the IUD-associated problems.

When the IUD is not removed, the woman has less than a 50% chance of delivering a live infant, compared to at least a 70% chance in normal pregnancies. Even if circumstances permit the removal of the device, the chance of a spontaneous abortion will be in the range of 25%–30% (twice the normal rate). A pregnant woman with an IUD also faces a risk of premature delivery that is as much as four times greater than in normal pregnancies.

The most serious possible outcome of a pregnancy with an IUD in place is intrauterine sepsis. Infection within the uterine cavity can cause serious morbidity and even maternal death. Indeed, in cases of spontaneous abortion, there is an estimated 25 times greater risk of mortality with this event if the IUD remains in the pregnant uterus. The clinician and the client should understand that the *overall* risk of this mortality is very low, but these figures are an important guide for judging prudent clinical practice.

Intrauterine sepsis associated with a pregnancy in an IUD user usually occurs in the second trimester. It may have rapid onset without localizing signs and can proceed to catastrophic infection and death. Fever is often the first symptom, with uterine dysfunction and spontaneous abortion occuring in only the latter part of the disease process. This differs from *septic abortion*, in which uterine bleeding and cramping generally *precede* the onset of fever.

Because intrauterine sepsis associated with pregnancy can begin and advance so rapidly without obvious symptoms, all pregnant women with an IUD in place should be kept under close surveillance and must be seen at once if fever should develop. If intrauterine infection is thought to have become established, immediate massive antibiotic therapy and emptying of the uterus are mandatory.

Cases of intrauterine sepsis during pregnancy related to IUD use have been reported with all commonly used devices. *All* types of IUDs should therefore be removed from the pregnant uterus during the first trimester if the string is visible, and therapeutic abortion should be offered otherwise.

Ectopic pregnancy.   It has been noted that the IUD use seems to be associated with a higher incidence of ectopic pregnancy (pregnancy developing outside the uterus). A causal relationship was sought. New research indicates that this assumption is inaccurate.

The Women's Health Study, a large survey of U.S. hospital data, found that all current contraceptive users are less likely to have an ectopic pregnancy than nonusers. Women using an IUD or a diaphragm have 40% *less* risk, and oral contraceptive users have one-tenth the risk. This *protective* effect of IUD use against ectopic pregnancy is a remarkably different concept from previous assumptions. This effect only seems to last for the first 2 years of IUD use, however, after which the risk of ectopic pregnancy returns to that of nonusers, but does *not* exceed normal rates.

The presence of an IUD in the uterus does increase the likelihood that *if* an accidental pregnancy occurs, it will be ectopic. Approximately 5% of all pregnancies among IUD users are ectopic, compared to an estimated 0.5% occurrence of ectopic gestations among pregnant women not using contraception. Despite this higher comparative risk, the incidence of ectopic pregnancy in IUD users is still very low—an estimated 0.5 per 1000 woman-years of use. Apparently, the increased proportion of ectopic pregnancy among IUD users results from the fact that IUDs prevent intrauterine pregnancies better than they do tubal pregnancies. If an accidental pregnancy does occur, therefore, it is more likely to be an ectopic gestation.

Table 3-11. **Symptoms of Ectopic Pregnancy.**
• Abnormal uterine bleeding • Pelvic pain or tenderness (especially after first year of IUD use) • Palpable adnexal mass or tenderness • Recent spotting

Women who have had one ectopic pregnancy have an increased risk of having another in the remaining fallopian tube. Since IUD use is not as protective against ectopic pregnancy as other contraceptive methods, these women should *not* use an IUD unless no other available method is acceptable.

Family planning providers must be keenly aware of the possibility of ectopic pregnancy among IUD users. An ectopic pregnancy could ruin the utility of the affected fallopian tube and, if left untreated, could result in extensive intraabdominal bleeding. One review of this subject noted that the diagnosis of ectopic pregnancy was initially unsuspected in 75% of the cases, and the patient's symptoms of unusual bleeding and cramps were often attributed to the IUD alone. An aid to correctly diagnosing ectopic pregnancy is the fact that most IUD problems—bleeding, pain, expulsion and pregnancy—tend to occur during the first year of use, whereas approximately two-thirds of the ectopic pregnancies in IUD users occur *after* 1 year of use. Nevertheless, regardless of the duration of IUD use, any woman who experiences abnormal bleeding or abdominal pain should be immediately examined for the possibility of ectopic pregnancy (Table 3-11).

Pelvic inflammatory disease. The occurrence of pelvic inflammatory disease (PID) is the complication of greatest concern with the use of IUDs. Estimates for the incidence of pelvic infection in IUD users range widely, depending on the experimental model, the definitions used, and the population evaluated. In the past, researchers conducting large-scale clinical studies tended to view PID as a relatively minor complication of IUD use. Researchers and providers today recognize the importance of this hazard.

The evaluation of PID among IUD users is hampered by imprecise definitions and diagnostic criteria. Pelvic inflammatory disease is not one but a group of several conditions, and different practitioners have different standards for identifying the disease on examination. Furthermore, few research studies have controlled for similar standards in client screening (to eliminate those prone to PID) and insertion technique (which, if done incorrectly, could contribute to infection). A Swedish study of women suspected of having PID confirmed the diagnosis by laparoscopy (direct visualization through the abdomen) in only *two-thirds* of the cases. Finally, even the occurrence of PID in the general population is not precisely known; estimates vary by an order of magnitude—from 1 to 20 per 1000 women per year. This makes a meaningful estimate of the relative risk in IUD users very difficult.

Nevertheless, a pattern has begun to emerge from the dozens of studies conducted on this question: when "objective" criteria of PID diagnosis are used, such as PID requiring hospitalization or PID confirmed through laparoscopy, the relative risk for IUD users is about 1.6 times that of nonusers. When broader criteria are used, such as suggestive symptoms including fever, the relative risk in IUD users is three to seven times that of nonusers. The most accurate statement that can be made at the present time is that there *is* an association between IUD use and pelvic inflammatory disease, but the relative risk cannot be estimated.

Removal for pelvic infection (both major and minor) accounts for up to 6% of IUD discontinuation in large-scale clinical studies. Apparently both nonmedicated and medicated devices are associated with similar rates of PID. It appears that the increased risk of PID does persist for up to a year after IUD removal, but it is not clear whether the risk is related to length of use.

Although providers cannot accurately predict which clients will develop PID, several risk factors for pelvic infection have been identified besides IUD use. Young nulliparous women with multiple sex partners are at the highest risk of PID. Thus nulliparity is recommended as a contraindication to IUD use, especially since pelvic infection can theoretically lead to tubal damage and infertility. But the risk of PID in older parous women is likely to be very low.

No research study has been able to prove that IUD use *causes* PID, and indeed such a mechanism can only be guessed at. It has been established that bacteria are frequently introduced into the uterine cavity at the time of IUD insertion. Fortunately, the endometrium has a remarkable self-cleansing property, and bacterial cultures from the uterus have been found to become negative within 30 days of IUD insertion. It is postulated that the causative organisms for PID may gain entry into the uterine cavity at the time of men-

struation or intercourse, penetrating the normally protective cervical mucus by way of the IUD string. If the IUD has embedded in the
myometrium, this may provide a site for bacterial invasion.

The causative organism of PID in IUD users may be gonococci
but more commonly is a normal vaginal contaminant such as chlamydia, actinomyces, *Escherichia coli*, mycoplasma, beta strepto-
cocci, bacteroides, or peptostreptococci. Table 3-12 summarizes the
differential diagnosis between gonococcal and nongonococcal pelvic
infection. Chlamydia is likely to be a frequent cause of IUD-associated PID. Researchers in the United States and Sweden have recently documented an "epidemic" of chlamydial infections. Unfortunately, chlamydia is difficult to culture.

A small proportion of pelvic infections found in IUD users will
be caused by actinomyces. The diagnosis is nearly impossible to
confirm, but "actinomyces-like" organisms may be seen on the Pap
smear. If the client has symptoms of infection and actinomyces-like
organisms are found on the Pap smear, the IUD should be removed
and penicillin begun. But actinomyces is a normal vaginal organism, so that if the client is asymptomatic, the IUD can be left in
place and follow-up Pap smears taken. Some studies have implied
that an actinomyces infection is more likely in users of nonmedicated devices, perhaps because of a bacteriostatic action by copper;
therefore, nonmedicated devices perhaps should be removed every
few years. This practice is *not* justified by current research evidence.

	Table 3-12. Distinguishing Gonococcal and Nongonococcal Pelvic Infection.	
	Gonococcal	**Nongonococcal**
Onset	Acute, sudden	Not acute, insidious
Pain	Acute	Vague, may come and go
Bleeding	Usually associated with menstruation—heavier and longer	Usually intermenstrual irregularities
Fever	Present, can be high	Usually not present, low if present
Treatment	Penicillin; tetracycline	Tetracycline; erythromycin
	Adapted from Gromko, 1980.	

In developing countries, PID may be more prevalent than in developed countries and its causes vary. Gonorrhea is widespread in Africa, where it is estimated to be the cause of up to 50% of the high infertility rates; however it is not an important cause of PID in India, for instance, where genital tuberculosis is more responsible. Where PID is more prevalent, IUD complication rates may be higher. This is the opposite of oral contraceptive complications, which are suspected to be lower in developing countries, where circulatory disease is less prevalent.

In cases of serious pelvic infection in IUD users, the device should be removed immediately and antibiotic therapy begun. Penicillin or tetracycline are still the antibiotics of choice in treating gonococcal PID; tetracycline or erythromycin is recommended for nongonococcal infections.

The infection may spread beyond the uterus, affecting the rest of the reproductive system and pelvic cavity. Women with PID have 10 times the risk of developing an ectopic pregnancy. Rarely, the infection can lead to development of an abscess involving both the tube and the ovary (tuboovarian abscess). This condition can harm future fertility, and if the abscess ruptures, widespread intraabdominal infection may result. The symptoms of this condition generally include several weeks of vague lower abdominal pain, dyspareunia (painful or difficult intercourse), and pelvic tenderness, with the subsequent development of fever and abscess. Immediate removal of the IUD is recommended if these symptoms occur, and appropriate antibiotic treatment should be initiated. Surgery may be necessary to remove the abscess.

If a tuboovarian abscess develops in an IUD user, it may be more likely to be unilateral (one-sided) than most abscesses found in the general population. A unilateral abscess, which affects only one tube and one ovary, offers the hope that fertility can be preserved with the undamaged side.

Despite the potential seriousness of pelvic inflammatory disease, permanent infertility is fortunately infrequent. It is not possible to state the probability of infertility developing in IUD users. But it has been estimated that 5%–10% of all IUD users have pelvic infections and that about 20% of them will become infertile. Therefore, only 1%–2% of those women *who discontinue IUD use in order to become pregnant* will fail to do so. For older multiparous women who are not likely to develop PID, therefore, the threat to their future fertility posed by IUD use is extremely low.

Table 3-13. Symptoms of Pelvic Inflammatory Disease.
• Purulent vaginal discharge • Fever (100.4°F) • Abnormal uterine bleeding • Lower abdominal pain • Painful intercourse • Palpable pelvic mass

There is controversy among practitioners regarding the need to remove an IUD if the woman develops *mild* pelvic infection. Some authors recommend that the IUD be left in place and the woman treated with antibiotics, whereas others believe that immediate IUD removal is mandatory so that the uterus no longer harbors a foreign body that may aggravate the infection. It seems prudent to conclude that early IUD removal with antibiotic treatment represents the safest approach. Of course, the client must be offered alternate contraception.

The woman may want to continue using the IUD despite mild pelvic infection, or her need and desire for preventing pregnancy may be strong and the use of another means of contraception unlikely. In this case, the device should be left in place, appropriate antibiotics administered, and the woman monitored carefully.

If a woman is about to undergo gynecological surgery with an IUD left in place, prophylactic antibiotics should be administered.

The risk of serious infection can be reduced by proper client screening, sterile prepackaging or in-clinic sterilization of the IUD, careful antiseptic measures, and sterile technique for insertion. Any woman who has had a recent septic abortion, postpartum endometritis, or any suspected pelvic inflammation should not have an IUD inserted for at least 3 months.

Family planning personnel must be aware of the dangers of PID. Purulent vaginal discharge, fever, abnormal bleeding, lower abdominal pain, or dyspareunia may be warning symptoms of developing or chronic pelvic infection and must be treated (Table 3-13). Any woman with these complaints should be seen promptly, and have the IUD removed and undergo antibiotic therapy if pelvic infection is suspected. If the patient is found to have an abnormal pelvic mass, this may be the result of a tuboovarian abscess, ovarian cyst, or ectopic pregnancy, and further diagnostic and therapeutic measures must be undertaken without delay.

CONCLUSION

After a detailed discussion of the possible complications of IUD use and their management, the risks and benefits need to be balanced once again, and the status of IUDs as a method of "second choice" should be reconsidered. The majority of women who have an IUD inserted experience neither side-effects nor complications. Most of the problems occurring in IUD users are self-limiting—they will either disappear within a few months or will stop as soon as the IUD is removed. The incidence of side-effects such as bleeding or pain falls sharply with duration of IUD use. Expulsion and perforation are directly related to the care taken at insertion, proper device selection, and the skill of clinician.

Virtually no IUD complications are life-threatening. Pregnancy—whether intrauterine or ectopic—is a serious but rare event that can be handled safely with proper management. The only side-effect of IUD use that can linger is PID with especially serious potential implications for nulliparous women. But the odds of serious PID occurring in older IUD users with no other PID risk factors are very low. For such women who may be seeking a coitally independent contraceptive method, IUDs can be an excellent choice.

Selected Readings

Anonymous: IUDs and actinomyces-like organisms. Lancet 1: 321, February 7, 1981

Ansari AH: Diagnosis and management of intrauterine device with missing tail. Obstetrics and Gynecology 44(5): 727, November 1974

Berger GS, Edelman DA, Reginie SJ: Patients responses to IUD insertion. International Journal of Gynecology and Obstetrics 14(2): 147, 1976

Berggren GG, Vaillant HW, Garnier H: Lippes Loop insertion by midwives in healthy and chronically ill women in rural Haiti. American Journal of Public Health 64(7): 719, July 1974

Bernard, RP: Factors governing IUD performance. American Journal of Public Health 61(3): 559, March 1971

Black TRL, Goldstruck ND, Spence A: Post-coital intrauterine device insertion—a further evaluation. Contraception 22(6): 653, December 1980

Boria MC, Gordon M: Complications from intrauterine devices: Postpartum and postabortal insertions. Journal of Reproductive Medicine 14(6): 251, June 1975

Burkman RT: Association between intrauterine device and pelvic inflammatory disease. Obstetrics and Gynecology 57(3): 269, March 1981

Cates W, Ory HW, Rochat RW, et al: The intrauterine device and deaths from spontaneous abortion. New England Journal of Medicine 295(21): 1155, November 18, 1976

Cates W, Grimes DA, Ory HW, et al: Publicity and the public health: The elimination of IUD-related abortion deaths. Family Planning Perspectives 9(2): 138, May/June 1977

Charles D: Infections in obstetrics and gynecology. Major Problems in Obstetrics and Gynecology (vol 12). Philadelphia, Saunders, 1980, pp 30, 77, 206

Curtis EM, Pine L: Actinomyces in the vaginas of women with and without intrauterine contraceptive devices. American Journal of Obstetrics and Gynecology 140(8): 880, August 15, 1981

Davies AJ, Anderson ABM, Turnbull AC: Reduction by Naproxen of excessive menstrual bleeding in women using intrauterine devices. Obstetrics and Gynecology 57(1): 74, January 1981

Dingfelder JR: Primary dysmenorrhea treatment with prostaglandin inhibitors; a review. American Journal of Obstetrics and Gynecology 140(8): 874, August 15, 1981

Drill VA, O'Brien FB: Cervical and uterine perforations by copper-containing intrauterine contraceptive devices. American Journal of Obstetrics and Gynecology 122(4): 535, June 15, 1975

Duguid HLD, Parratt D, Traynor R: Actinomyces-like organisms in cervical smears from women using intrauterine contraceptive devices. British Medical Journal 281: 534, 1980

Edelman D, Berger GS, Keith L: Intrauterine Devices and Their Complications. Boston, Hall, 1979, 263 pp

Edelman DA, Goldsmith A, Shelton JD: Postpartum contraception. International Journal of Gynecology and Obstetrics 19: 305, August 1981

Eisinger SH: Second trimester spontaneous abortion, the IUD, and infection. American Journal of Obstetrics and Gynecology 124(4): 393, February 15, 1976

Erkola R, Liukko P: Intrauterine device and ectopic pregnancy. Contraception 16(6): 569, December 1977

Foreman H, Stadel BV, Schlesselman S: Intrauterine device usage and fetal loss. Obstetrics and Gynecology 58(6): 669, December 1981

Gentile GP, Siegler AM: The misplaced or missing IUD. Obstetrical and Gynecological Survey 32(10): 627, 1977

Ginsburg DS, Stern JC, Hamod KA, et al: Tubo-ovarian abscess—a retrospective review. American Journal of Obstetrics and Gynecology 138(7): 1042, December 1980

Gobeaux-Castadot MJ, Boria MC, Chervanak FA, et al: Five year clinical experience with the Copper-7 intrauterine contraceptive devices. International Journal of Gynecology and Obstetrics 19: 181, June 1981

Goldsmith A: Intrauterine devices in the immediate postabortal period, in Holtrop HR, Waife RS, Bustamente W, et al (eds): New Developments in Fertility Regulation. Chestnut Hill, MA, The Pathfinder Fund, 1976, p 182

Gosden C, Steel J, Ross A, Springbett A: Intrauterine contraceptive devices in diabetic women. Lancet 1: 530, March 6, 1982

Gromko L: Intrauterine devices. Nurse Practitioner 5: 17, July/August 1980

Guillebaud J: IUD and congenital malformation. British Medical Journal 1: 1016, 1976

Guillebaud J: Management of bleeding problems with intrauterine devices. Fertility and Contraception 1(1): 9, January 1977

Guillebaud J, Bonnar J, Morehead J, et al: Menstrual blood-loss with intrauterine devices. Lancet 1: 387, February 21, 1976

Hager WD, Douglas B, Majmudar B, et al: Pelvic colonization with actinomyces in women using intrauterine contraceptive devices. American Journal of Obstetrics and Gynecology 135: 680, November 1979

Hallatt JG: Ectopic pregnancy associated with the intrauterine device: A study of seventy cases. American Journal of Obstetrics and Gynecology 125(6): 754, July 15, 1976

Hatcher RA: A case against the use of IUDs for teenagers. Advances in Planned Parenthood 15(2): 48, 1980

Hefnawi F, Kandil D, Askalani H, et al: Influence of the copper IUD and the Lippes Loop on sperm migration in the human cervical mucus. Contraception 11(5): 541, May 1975

Hefnawi F, Segal SJ (eds): Analysis of Intrauterine Contraception. Amsterdam, North-Holland, 1975, 490 pp

Huber SC, Piotrow PT, Orlans FB, et al: IUDs reassessed: A decade of experience. Population Reports B(2), Washington, DC, George Washington University, January 1975

Huggins GR: Contraceptive use and subsequent fertility. Fertility and Sterility 28(6): 603, June 1977

Jacobson L: Differential diagnosis of acute pelvic inflammatory disease. American Journal of Obstetrics and Gynecology 138(7): 1006, December 1980

Jain AK: Safety and effectiveness of IUDs. Contraception 11(3): 293, March 1975

Kahn HS, Tyler CW: An association between the Dalkon Shield and complicated pregnancies among women hospitalized for IUCD-related disorders. American Journal of Obstetrics and Gynecology 125(1): 83, May 1, 1976

Kahn HS, Tyler CW: Mortality associated with use of IUDs. Journal of the American Medical Association 234(1): 57, October 6, 1975

Kamal I, Ohoneim M, Tallaat M, et al: Pregnancies in the presence of copper intrauterine devices. International Journal of Gynecology and Obstetrics 14(4): 341, 1976

Kaye BM, Reaney BV, Kaye DL, et al: Long-term safety and use-effectiveness of intrauterine devices. Fertility and Sterility 28(9): 937, September 1977

King K: The Chlamydia epidemic. Journal of the American Medical Association 245(17): 1718, May 1, 1981

Laes E, Lehtovirta P, Weintraub D, et al: Early puerperal insertions of Copper T-200. Contraception 11(3): 289, March 1975

Larsson B, Hamberger L: Insertion of Copper 7 IUD in connection with induced abortions during the first trimester. Contraception 12(1): 69, July 1975

Law RG: Problems related to the recognition of intrauterine contraceptive devices by ultrasound. British Journal of Family Planning 6: 35, July 1980

Lippes J: IUD-related hospitalization and mortality. Journal of the American Medical Association 235(10): 1001, March 8, 1976

Lippes J, Malik T, Tatum HJ: The postcoital Copper T. Advances in Planned Parenthood 11(1): 24, 1976

Mandouvalos H, Gouskos A: Germicidal effect of pure electrolytic Copper on the gonococcus. Contraceptive Delivery Systems 2(3): 225, July 1981

Measham AR, Villegas A: Comparison of continuation rates of intrauterine devices. Obstetrics and Gynecology 48(3): 336, September 1976

Muir DG, Belsey MA: Pelvic inflammatory disease and its consequences in the developed world. American Journal of Obstetrics and Gynecology 138(7): 913, December 1980

Newton JR, Reading AE: The effects of psychological preparation on pain at intrauterine device insertion. Contraception 16(5): 523, November 1977

Oakley N, Stanton SL: Contraception and diabetes. British Journal of Family Planning 8: 55, 1982

Orlans FB: Copper IUDs: Performance to date. Population Reports B(1), Washington, DC, George Washington University, December 1973

Ory HW: Ectopic pregnancy and intrauterine contraceptive devices: new perspectives. Obstetrics and Gynecology 57(2): 137, February 1981

Oster G, Salgo MP: The copper intrauterine device and its mode of action. New England Journal of Medicine 293(9): 432, August 28, 1975

Pastene L, Rivera M, Zipper J, et al: IUD insertions by midwives: Five years' experience in Santiago, Chile. International Journal of Gynecology and Obstetrics 15(1): 84, 1977

Piotrow Pt, Rinehart W, Schmidt JC: IUDs—update on safety, effectiveness and research. Population Reports B(3). Baltimore, Johns Hopkins University, May 1979, 52 pp

Potts M, Speidel JJ, Kessel E: Relative risks of various means of fertility control when used in less-developed countries, in Sciarra JJ, Zatuchni GI, Speidel JJ (eds): Risks, Benefits and Controversies in Fertility Control. Hagerstown, MD, Harper & Row, 1978, p 28

Reading AE, Newton JR: Psychological factors in IUD use—a review. Journal of Biosocial Science 9: 317, 1977

Rees E: The treatment of pelvic inflammatory disease. American Journal of Obstetrics and Gynecology 138(7): 1042, December 1980

Rivera R, Almonte H, Arreola M, et al: The use of different hormonal contraceptives and IUDs in anemic women—a six month follow up. Advances in Planned Parenthood 15(2): 56, 1980

Rivera R, de Tanco MU, de Velasquez G, et al: Indigenous paramedical personnel in family planning in rural Durango, Mexico. Pathpaper No. 3, Chestnut Hill, MA, The Pathfinder Fund, June 1978

Roy S, Shaw ST: Role of prostaglandins in IUD-associated uterine bleeding—effect of a prostaglandin synthetase inhibitor (Ibuprofen). Obstetrics and Gynecology 58: 101, 1981

Senanayake P, Kramer DG: Contraception and the etiology of pelvic inflammatory disease: New perspectives. American Journal of Obstetrics and Gynecology 138(7): 852, December 1980

Senanayake P, Kramer DG: Contraception and pelvic inflammatory disease. IPPF Medical Bulletin 16(2): 3, April 1982

Snowden R: Copper IUCDs and the pregnancy rate. British Journal of Family Planning 6: 104, 1981

Snowden R, Eckstein P, Hawkins D: Social and medical factors in the use and effectiveness of IUDs. Journal of Biosocial Science 5: 31, 1973

Tatum HJ, Schmidt FH: Contraception and sterilization practices and extrauterine pregnancy: A realistic perspective. Fertility and Sterility 28(4): 407, April 1977

Tatum HJ, Schmidt FH, Jain AK: Management and outcome of pregnancies associated with the Copper T intrauterine device. American Journal of Obstetrics and Gynecology 126(7): 869, December 1, 1976

Tatum HJ, Schmidt FH, Philips D, et al: The Dalkon Shield controversy: Structural and bacteriologic studies of IUD tails. Journal of the American Medical Association 231(7): 711, Februrary 17, 1975

Taylor ES, McMillan JH, Green BE, et al: The intrauterine device and tubo-ovarian abscess. American Journal of Obstetics and Gynecology 123(4): 338, October 15, 1975

Thiery M: Immediate postpartum insertion of IUDs. International Planned Parenthood Foundation Medical Bulletin 15(3), June 1981

Thiery M, Van der Pas H, Delbeke L, et al: Immediate postpartum insertion of a copper-wired IUD, the ML Cu250. British Journal of Obstetrics and Gynecology 86: 654, August 1979

Thiery M, Van Kets H, Kurz K, et al: Intrauterine contraceptive devices for diabetic women. Lancet 2: 883, October 16, 1982

Tietze C: New estimates of mortality associated with fertility control. Family Planning Perspectives 9(2): 74, March/April 1977

Tietze C, Lewit S: Evaluation of intrauterine devices: Ninth progress report of the Cooperative Statistical Program. Studies in Family Planning No. 55, July 1970

Tyrer LB: The Copper-7 and postcoital contraceptives. Advances in Planned Parenthood 15(3): 111, 1980

Valicenti JF, Pappas AA, Graber CD, et al: Detection and Prevalence of IUD-associated actinomyces colonization and related morbidity: A prospective study of 69,925 cervical smears. Journal of the American Medical Association 247(8): 1149, February 26, 1982

Van Os W, Bomert I, Rhemrev P, et al: Evaluation of the combined Multiload copper intrauterine device (MlCu 250). Fertility and Sterility 28(3): 291, March 1977

Van Santen MR, Haspels AA: Interception by post-coital IUD insertion. Contraceptive Delivery Systems 2(3): 189, July 1981

Vessey M, Lawless M, Yeates D: Efficacy of different contraceptive methods. Lancet 1: 841, April 10, 1982

Westrom L: Incidence, prevalence, and trends of acute pelvic inflammatory disease and its consequences in industrialized countries. American Journal of Obstetrics and Gynecology 138(7): 880, December 1980

White MK, Brooks JB, Strauss L, et al: Current practice concerning time of IUD insertion. International Planned Parenthood Foundation Medical Bulletin 11(6): 1, December 1977

Williams P, et al: Septic abortion in women using intrauterine devices. British Medical Journal 4: 263, November 1, 1975

World Health Organization: Interval IUD insertion in parous women: a randomized multicentre comparative trial of the Lippes Loop D, TCu220C and the Copper 7. Contraception 26(1): 1, July 1982

Wortman J: Training nonphysicians in family planning services. Population Reports J(6), Washington, DC, George Washington University, September 1975

Wright NH, Sujpluem C, Rosenfield AG, et al: Nurse-midwife insertion of the Copper T in Thailand: Performance, acceptance and programmatic effects. Studies in Family Planning 8(9): 237, September 1977

Zakin D, Stern WZ, Rosenblatt R: Complete and partial uterine perforation and embedding following insertion of intrauterine devices II—diagnostic methods, prevention and management. Obstetrical and Gynecological Survey 36(8): 401, August 1981

Barrier Methods

4

Barrier methods are the oldest means of contraception and have been in use for centuries. As early as the 19th century B.C., Egyptian papyri described the use of vaginal tampons coated with crocodile dung, oils, honey, and other ingredients to create a spermicidal effect. Halves of various fruit skins were used in much the same way as diaphragms or cervical caps are today. Penile sheaths—forerunners of condoms—probably date back to Egyptian times. Over the centuries, the concept of barrier contraception has changed little: to prevent pregnancy by blocking sperm from entering the uterus, either mechanically or chemically.

Until recently the mechanical and chemical barrier methods were the only effective means of contraception available and thus were widely used. With the development of oral contraceptives and modern IUDs in the 1960s, the popularity of barrier contraception plummeted since these new methods were highly effective, more aesthetically appealing, and not coitus-related. In the United States, for example, the use of diaphragms fell by 60% between 1955 and 1965. This trend was further intensified by the introduction of improved sterilization techniques in the 1970s.

Renewed interest in barrier methods has resulted from concerns about the side-effects and safety of oral contraceptives and IUDs and the recognition that they are not necessarily the best methods for all individuals. Although the cardiovascular dangers of oral contraceptives now appear to apply almost exclusively to women over 35 who smoke, the association between pelvic infections and IUDs is a very important concern for younger couples who have not completed childbearing.

131

Barrier methods offer an alternative to prolonged pill or IUD use for women who delay childbearing into their late 20s and early to mid-30s. The development and legal availability of safe abortion techniques providing a backup should barrier contraceptives fail have also contributed to renewed use of barrier methods.

Family planning providers are reassessing barrier contraception and recognizing the advantages and diversity of these simple methods. For many family planning clients, the barrier methods have special appeal because they do not act systemically and thus have fewer side-effects. In addition, from a public health standpoint, barrier contraceptives offer a major advantage over other family planning methods: they help to reduce the spread of sexually transmitted diseases and apparently also provide protection against pelvic inflammatory disease (PID).

INDICATIONS

The barrier methods are indicated for any client who desires safe, reversible contraception. The barrier user should understand that the somewhat lower effectiveness rate of barrier methods means a greater risk of having an unwanted pregnancy when compared with using oral contraceptives or IUDs. Nevertheless, barrier methods may be particularly useful when:

- Intercourse is infrequent.
- "Over-the-counter" availability is important (such as with adolescents).
- A temporary contraceptive method is needed between pregnancies or before a first pregnancy.
- Both partners want to share in the responsibility for contraception.
- The woman is older and oral contraceptives are contraindicated.
- Couples in some cultures may better relate to the concept of barrier methods that are similar to traditional methods.
- No other contraceptive methods are available or acceptable.

There will always be couples for whom barrier methods are the most appropriate, acceptable, or available. Family planning providers must remember that the use of *any* safe and reasonably effective contraceptive method is better than none at all and can make an important contribution to maternal and child health.

EFFECTIVENESS

The contraceptive effectiveness of barrier methods depends almost entirely on how consistently and properly the client uses them. This makes the calculation of effectiveness rates very difficult. As a consequence, the *theoretical effectiveness* rate is distinguished from the *use effectiveness* rate. Theoretical effectiveness of barrier methods means how well the spermicide, condom, diaphragm, or combination thereof should work in preventing sperm from fertilizing the ovum. This rate is usually estimated to be very high. Use effectiveness tries to estimate the likelihood of the user being able to properly insert the diaphragm, apply the spermicide, use condoms without leakage, and so on. These estimated rates are based on clinical trials studying actual users' success in avoiding pregnancy over time, and they generally have been found to be lower. Use effectiveness rates also vary considerably, and the key to successful use is client motivation and understanding (see below). Theoretical and use effectiveness rates for the barrier methods are shown in Figure 4-1; these rates are discussed in detail in each section of this chapter.

Although barrier methods should not be unfairly deemphasized by a provider as they have been in the past, both provider and client should remember that effectiveness is not merely a theoretical con-

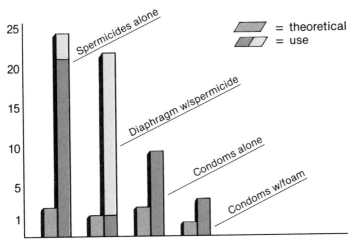

Figure 4-1. *Comparative theoretical and use effectiveness rates for barrier methods of contraception, showing estimated pregnancy rates for 100 woman-years of method use. Compare this figure with Figure 2-1. (Adapted from Hatcher et al., 1980; Vessey et al., 1982; and others.)*

cept. Lower effectiveness means a greater chance of contraceptive failure; contraceptive failure means an unwanted pregnancy. When any contraceptive method is judged, the consequences of failure must be understood and the physical and psychosocial risks of unwanted pregnancy considered.

Attitudes and Motivation

There are many ways to improve use effectiveness of barrier methods. The first step is *provider attitude*. Family planning clinics that do not commit sufficient resources to stocking, resupplying, promoting, and explaining barrier methods are setting up obstacles to their use. The attitude of individual providers is very important when the client seeks assistance in making a contraceptive choice. Family planning personnel sometimes discourage barrier method use in favor of the more modern "scientific" methods. Busy practitioners may deemphasize barrier method options because of the time required to fully explain their proper use. All things being equal, a client who visits a clinic that objectively offers barrier methods as an integral service will be more likely to consider them. On the other hand, clients will reject barrier methods if they perceive negative attitudes about them from clinic personnel. The provider must inspire confidence in the method chosen so that it is used regularly and consistently.

Client motivation is an equally critical prerequisite to the successful use of barrier methods. User characteristics that lead to consistent and highly effective use should be considered by provider and client when making the contraceptive choice. Both partners should be motivated to avoid pregnancy and must have agreed between themselves about contraceptive responsibility. They also must be able to adapt their sexual relationship in a comfortable way for proper barrier method use. They need to *want* to use the method they choose and accept the steps necessary to use it properly. With barrier methods, successful use will require more discipline.

Finally, proper *client education* will greatly increase the chances that use of barrier methods will effectively prevent an unwanted pregnancy. A clear understanding of how the method works will improve user confidence and actual method effectiveness. For example, the knowledge that some spermatozoa are still alive in the vagina after the penis has been withdrawn underscores the need for leaving a diaphragm in place at least 6 hours after intercourse. In each section of this chapter, detailed suggestions are given for client education.

The motivation and education process does not end when the method is first chosen. Checking on continuing client motivation and reinforcement of client understanding about method function are important components of the follow-up process.

DIAPHRAGMS

The diaphragm is a dome-shaped latex cup used with spermicidal cream or jelly to create an effective contraceptive barrier (Figure 4-2). The modern diaphragm was developed 100 years ago, but methods based on the same principle have been a primary means of contraception for centuries. It is known that by the 18th century, women in various countries used molded beeswax, opium, oiled paper, half lemons, and other materials to create crude vaginal contraceptive devices similar in shape to the diaphragm.

The modern diaphragm was invented in 1838, but not until the 1880s was it first publicized. A German physician using the pseudonym "Mensinga" described a pliable device held in place by a flexible metal rim that was incorporated into the rubber. The use of the diaphragm spread to Holland and later to England, where it became known as the "Dutch cap." During the 1920s, the Holland-Rantos Company began manufacturing diaphragms in the United States.

Selection

In recent years, the diaphragm has become increasingly popular as an alternative method of family planning among women who do not wish to use oral contraceptives or intrauterine devices (IUDs).

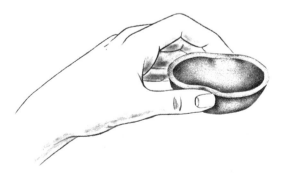

Figure 4-2. *The diaphragm.*

To use the diaphragm, the woman must coat it with spermicide and insert it into the vagina prior to intercourse. Held in place by a flexible spring molded into its rubber rim, the diaphragm fits across the upper vagina, covering the cervix and creating a partial physical barrier to sperm. The diaphragm is not, however, a spermtight barrier; its contraceptive effect results principally from its ability to hold a layer of spermicide directly against the cervix; therefore, the diaphragm should never be used without spermicidal cream or jelly.

Advantages and disadvantages. Diaphragm use involves clear advantages for some clients:

- Diaphragm use is generally free of known systemic effects or life-threatening complications; less serious side-effects are rare and limited mainly to allergic reactions.
- The diaphragm can be inserted up to 2 hours before intercourse and thus need not interrupt sexual foreplay.
- Since the diaphragm occludes the cervix, when used during menstruation it will capture the menstrual blood, making intercourse during the period more acceptable to some couples.
- Spermicidal creams and jellies used with a diaphragm have some bacteria-killing effects and can decrease the risk of sexually transmitted infection.

Despite these advantages, limitations to diaphragm use do exist:

- Medical skills are needed for examination, fitting, and instruction.
- The diaphragm is relatively cumbersome and messy to use. As it necessitates far more manipulation of the genitals than any other barrier method, it may be unacceptable for some people.
- It must be used faithfully and carefully with each coital act, requiring considerable contraceptive motivation and planning.
- A degree of privacy for insertion and removal is considered necessary by some women. In developing countries, a ready source of water is needed for washing the device after use.

Contraindications. Diaphragm fitting should not be attempted at all if properly trained personnel are unavailable. Diaphragms are not advised for clients with known allergy to latex or spermicide or with physical abnormalities—such as uterine prolapse, poor vaginal muscle tone, cystocele, rectocele, severe and fixed uterine retroversion, vaginal fistulas, or vaginal septas—that may make diaphragm

Table 4-1.
Contraindications to Diaphragm Use.
• Allergy to latex or spermicides • Uterine prolapse, retroversion, cystocele, or rectocele • Poor vaginal muscle tone • Vaginal fistulas or septas • Client unable to insert the diaphragm correctly

fitting difficult or impossible (Table 4-1). A woman who cannot learn correct insertion techniques and cannot be assisted by her partner will also not be able to use a diaphragm. Sexual inexperience can be a contraindication to diaphragm use if the introitus is not adequately relaxed to allow user confidence and comfort.

Use

Fitting. What distinguishes the diaphragm from other barrier methods is that it must be properly fitted by a trained health worker. Fitting does not require a physician, though, and can be readily performed by a nurse, midwife, or other properly trained family planning provider.

Diaphragms vary both in size and according to the type of spring enclosed in the rim. The three types of springs are:

- Arcing spring: most widely used; inserts easily and is well tolerated by the majority of women
- Coil spring: especially suitable for nulliparous women
- Flat spring: rarely used; principally for women with poor muscle tone in the wall of either the bladder or rectum

Determining the proper diaphragm size is a key to effective use of this method. Diaphragm sizes are measured by the rim diameter, ranging from 50 to 105 mm. The most common sizes used are 75–85 mm, although nulliparous women may require a smaller size, usually 65 or 70.

During the bimanual pelvic examination, the practitioner will have looked for the anatomical abnormalities that contraindicate diaphragm use—especially uterine prolapse, extreme retroversion, or distortion of the vagina by either the bladder or the rectum (cystocele or rectocele).

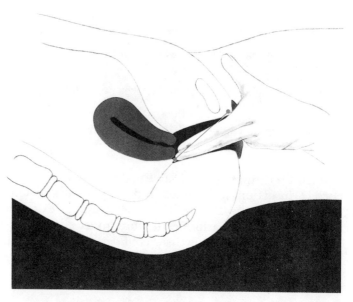

Figure 4-3. *Diaphragm fitting. The proper diaphragm diameter is selected by measuring the distance from the posterior vaginal fornia to the pubic bone.*

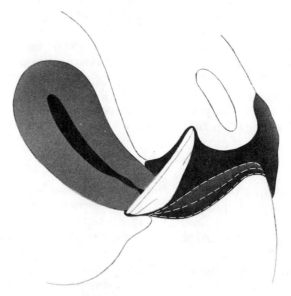

Figure 4-4. *Diaphragm fitting must consider the vaginal expansion that comes with sexual arousal.*

138

The practitioner then measures the diagonal length of the vagina from the pubic bone to the posterior vaginal fornix. The practitioner inserts the index and second fingers deep into the vagina until the tip of the second finger touches the posterior vaginal fornix. The point at which the index finger touches the pubic bone is noted and marked with a finger from the other hand. For comparison of this distance to the proper diaphragm diameter, one end of the diaphragm rim is placed on the tip of the second finger, and the other end of the rim is placed on the spot marked (Figure 4-3).

Fitting rings or sample diaphragms of various sizes are then used to verify appropriate fit, especially checking that the diaphragm will touch the lateral vaginal walls and that it will fit snugly. The provider's goal is to select the largest size that is comfortable for the woman, based on two factors: vaginal depth and width and vaginal muscle tone. The most common fitting error is selecting a size that is too small. Since the vagina expands during sexual arousal (Figure 4-4), a diaphragm that is too small may fail to maintain its position over the cervix. A diaphragm that is too large, however, may also cause problems such as uncomfortable pressure, abdominal pain, vaginal ulceration, or recurrent urinary tract infection.

Client instructions. Proper fitting is only half the provider's responsiblity to a diaphragm user; the woman must also be taught correct insertion and removal. Careful supportive instruction is crucial for effective use. The woman should be shown and allowed to practice insertion and removal at the time of the fitting. She should then be asked to return, within a week's time or less, with the device in place for checking of proper placement and fit. As she may be more relaxed during this second visit than during the initial fitting, decreased vaginal tone may be evident, necessitating change to a slightly larger diaphragm size.

The instructions the practitioner gives the new diaphragm user are extremely important for achieving effective contraception (Table 4-2). Key points to stress to the diaphragm user are:

1. A spermicide should always be used with the diaphragm. Clients can choose between contraceptive creams and jellies, which are equally effective for use with a diaphragm. This choice can be based on several factors: simple availability, preference for the consistency of one or the other, and individual variations in vaginal lubrication. Contraceptive creams are usually more viscous

Table 4-2.
Diaphragm Use: Client Instructions.

- Always use spermicidal cream or jelly.
- Coat inside of diaphragm dome and rim with spermicide.
- Fold diaphragm in half and insert into vagina, passing diaphragm back along the bottom wall of the vagina.
- Tuck back rim of diaphragm behind the cervix and tuck the front rim behind the pubic bone.
- Check placement to feel that cervix is covered.
- Insert diaphragm no more than 2 hours prior to intercourse.
- Leave in place for at least 6 hours after intercourse.
- If intercourse is repeated within 6 hours, leave the diaphragm in place and add an application of spermicide, using the plastic applicator.
- Remove diaphragm by sliding index finger between front rim and pubic bone, then gently pull foward and out.
- Rinse diaphragm with warm water—NO SOAP—then dry carefully and put back in case.
- Have fit rechecked annually, and after pregnancy, abortion, surgery, or weight change.

than jellies and thus provide less lubrication than do jellies. If a woman wishes additional vaginal lubrication, she might choose the contraceptive jelly over the cream. Some spermicidal manufacturers now offer contraceptive creams and jellies that are both odorless and tasteless.

2. The diaphragm dome should be held down like a cup and approximately one tablespoon of jelly or cream squeezed into the dome (Figure 4-5). Some of the spermicide should also be spread

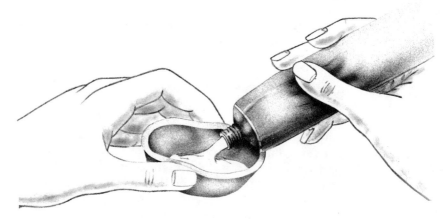

Figure 4-5. *The diaphragm must always be used with spermicide.*

around the inside of the rim to destroy sperm that might pass around the device.

3. The diaphragm should be inserted carefully and correctly. The woman should squeeze the opposite sides of the rim together with one hand so that the device folds in half. Spreading the labia with the other hand, she should insert the folded diaphragm into the vagina, passing it far back along the posterior vaginal wall until it comes to lie behind the cervix (Figure 4-6). Then she tucks the front part of the diaphragm up behind the pubic bone in the anterior vagina. In order for a woman to use the diaphragm correctly, it is important for her to understand the vaginal anatomy. A pelvic model can help the provider explain that the vagina passes backward, rather than vertically up her body. When inserting the diaphragm, the leading edge must therefore be directed horizontally if she is standing up, and vertically if she is lying down. The pelvic model will also help demonstrate the proper position of the diaphragm in relation to the cervix and reassure the woman that the diaphragm cannot "get lost" in her body.

4. The woman should insert the diaphragm immediately or no more than 2 hours before sexual intercourse.

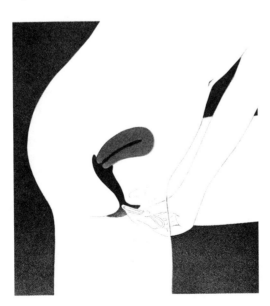

Figure 4-6. *The diaphragm can be inserted when the woman is standing with one leg raised or when she is reclining.*

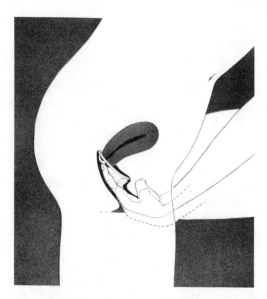

Figure 4-7. *The woman should check for proper placement by feeling the cervix through the diaphragm dome.*

5. After insertion, the woman should check that the diaphragm is properly placed (Figure 4-7). When it is in the correct position, its back rim lies below and behind the cervix in the posterior vagina, and the cervix can be felt through the rubber dome. The cervix is often described as feeling like the tip of the nose. The woman must be able to examine herself internally to identify the cervix and ensure proper diaphragm placement. The diaphragm is not a good contraceptive method for women who are averse to this type of self-examination.

6. The diaphragm must be left in place at least 6 hours after intercourse to allow complete spermicidal action. The diaphragm may be left in longer than 6 hours. If intercourse is repeated within 6 hours, an additional application of spermicide must be inserted vaginally by means of a plastic applicator. The diaphragm *should not* be removed at this time.

7. Proper removal and care are also important. To remove a diaphragm, the woman slides the index finger between the front rim of the diaphragm and the pubic bone to break the suction (Figure 4-8). While gently pulling down and out, being careful not to tear the rubber, she should bear down with her lower abdominal

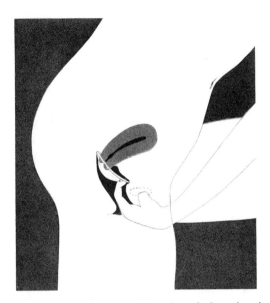

Figure 4-8. *The diaphragm should be removed gently and cleaned and stored properly.*

muscles. Once removed, the diaphragm should be washed with mild soap and water, rinsed, dried, and stored in the container it came in, away from intense heat if possible. It may be dusted with cornstarch prior to storage. Talcum and perfumed powders should not be used because of adverse side-effects for the client. Petroleum jelly (Vaseline) should not be used with a diaphragm as it can damage the rubber and reduce the life of the device. When properly cared for, a diaphragm should remain intact for several years, although it may become discolored. The woman should inspect her diaphragm regularly for holes or signs of deterioration, especially at the rim.

The diaphragm fit should be checked yearly and also after a pregnancy, abortion, pelvic surgery, or a weight change of 15 pounds or more. If diaphragm fitting occurs during lactation, the fit should be checked again 6 weeks after weaning or after normal menstruation resumes.

Side-effects. Although allergy to latex is rare, some diaphragm users develop vaginal irritation, swelling, or blistering, which most often are allergic reactions to the spermicidal cream or jelly.

Partners occasionally develop allergic reactions as well. Changing products will sometimes solve these problems. Some women may also report pelvic pain, vaginal ulceration, bladder pressure, urinary retention, urethral irritation, or recurrent cystitis or urethritis when the diaphragm is left in place the recommended 6 hours. These problems are likely the result of excessive rim pressure and can often be resolved by changing to a different diaphragm size or rim type. Diaphragm users should be advised to empty their bladders regularly while wearing the diaphragm. Often, this can mitigate some types of bladder discomfort.

Concerns were raised for the first time in 1981 about possible side-effects from the spermicides used in conjunction with the diaphragm (see page 153). Research is continuing to specifically identify these risks.

Effectiveness. The theoretical effectiveness of the diaphragm with spermicide is 98%, or 2 pregnancies per 100 woman-years. Studies of the actual use effectiveness of the diaphragm, however, show great variations in pregnancy rates. The use effectiveness rate most commonly estimated for the diaphragm is 87%, but in different studies this rate fluctuates from as high as 98% to as low as 77%. Well-motivated, careful users of the diaphragm, however, can achieve high levels of efficacy similar to the use effectiveness of IUDs and oral contraceptives.

Diaphragm failures more often result from problems with client motivation rather than from device defects. Failure rates are highest among new users—particularly those switching from more "convenient" methods—and also among persons wishing to delay rather than prevent conception. Failures also occur for behavioral reasons, such as not using spermicide or not inserting additional spermicide for repeated intercourse. Sometimes failures can occur if the diaphragm is displaced by coital motion.

The provider–client interaction is key to effective diaphragm use. Careful client selection, proper fitting, and thorough user instruction are all important. A correct fit alone will be of no value if the woman does not have the knowledge and motivation to use the diaphragm correctly. Diaphragm use necessitates more explanation and instruction than do the other barrier methods and requires a provider who communicates confidence and patience.

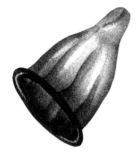 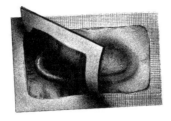

Figure 4-9. *The condom.*

CONDOMS

Condoms are thin sheaths that fit snugly over the penis and act as a mechanical barrier preventing ejaculated semen from entering the vagina (Figure 4-9). Much speculation abounds on the origin of condoms; penile sheaths shown in early Egyptian art may be the first record of this contraceptive. Condoms in various forms have been used for centuries as protection against pregnancy and sexually transmitted disease. The earliest condoms were made from linen or the membrane from animal intestines. The development of vulcanized rubber in the 19th century allowed the mass production and popularization of latex rubber condoms that are distributed worldwide today. Condoms are known by a host of popular names, such as "rubbers," "safes," "nirodh" (in India), "mechais" (in Thailand), and "prophylactics." Although used throughout the world, they are often not given appropriate recognition as a valuable nonclinical contraceptive method that meets two important public health goals: the prevention of unwanted pregnancies and the curbing of sexually transmitted diseases.

Selection

Most modern condoms are made from latex rubber and are either plain-end or reservoir-tipped to hold the ejaculate. To prevent friction, many condoms are lubricated with a glycol solution or a spermicide, or are coated with silicone. Condoms may also be ribbed or otherwise altered to provide added stimulation during intercourse. They are most often natural-colored but are now available in assorted colors. Natural skin condoms, made from sheep membrane, are available but expensive and constitute less than 1% of all condoms used. They are particularly useful for men who desire increased penile sensitivity or are allergic to rubber.

Advantages and disadvantages. Condom use offers many advantages:

- Condoms are highly effective when used consistently and correctly.
- Condom use permits active involvement and responsibility of the male partner.
- Because condoms are widely available and can be dispensed without medical examination or prescription, they can be used where no clinical services are available and can be distributed through preexisting commercial channels or community-based systems.
- Condoms offer better protection against sexually transmitted diseases than does any other contraceptive method.
- Cervical dysplasia (abnormal cells) may occur less frequently in women whose partners use condoms, and in women with cervical neoplasia (cancer), condom use may contribute to the regression of the disease.
- Condom use involves no health risks, medical complications, or side-effects, except for an occasional allergic reaction to rubber.
- Condom use eliminates vaginal discharge of semen after intercourse.
- Condoms are relatively inexpensive and convenient to use, carry, and throw away.
- Because condoms can decrease penile sensitivity, they can help to prolong intercourse.
- Lubricated condoms can be helpful to women who develop vaginal irritation from friction during intercourse.

Despite the many advantages to condoms, some problems do occur in conjunction with their use:

- Condoms require male responsibility and motivation, which may be lacking because of personal or cultural factors.

- Some couples complain of reduced sensations when condoms are used.
- Condoms can break, leading to contraceptive failure. Breakage is usually attributable to poor quality or incorrect use.
- Allergic reactions to rubber are rare but may occur; switching to natural skin condoms usually helps.
- Condoms must be put on after erection but prior to penetration. Many couples perceive this as a "disruption" of sexual foreplay. If they can make putting the condom on a *part* of foreplay, however, this disadvantage can be overcome.

Contraindications. There are virtually no contraindications to condom use, apart from allergy to rubber or difficulty in maintaining an erection.

Use

Client instruction. Although condoms provide a simple, effective contraceptive method, some instruction helps in their proper use. The man or his partner should be told to unroll the condom to full length over the erect penis before any vaginal contact (Figure 4-10). This is important because millions of sperm can be present in the preejaculatory fluid. If the condom is not reservoir-tipped, approximately 1.5 cm should be left free at the end to hold the ejaculate. Lubrication—water-soluble jelly, contraceptive foam, or saliva—can be applied if desired. After intercourse the man should withdraw his penis before it becomes flaccid, while holding the rim of the condom to prevent semen spilling in the vagina.

If semen has possibly spilled or if the condom is noted to be broken, a spermicidal preparation should be inserted into the vagina immediately. It is best to use a condom only once, but if necessary it can be washed with soap and water, tested for leaks, dried, and powdered with cornstarch and reused.

Side-effects. There are no known side-effects to condom use besides the occasional allergic reaction to latex.

Effectiveness. The theoretical effectiveness of condoms is 97%, but actual use effectiveness is estimated to be 90% (10 pregnancies per 100 woman-years). As with the other barrier methods, condom use effectiveness in some studies has been reported to be very high, especially when used with a spermicidal foam. Condoms and foam together have a theoretical effectiveness of 99% and use effectiveness of 95%. Since the effectiveness of condoms and foam together compares favorably with oral contraceptives and IUDs, the use of this combination can be encouraged as an attractive alternative when it is likely to be used properly and consistently.

One manufacturer in the United States and the United Kingdom is marketing a condom lubricated with the spermicide nonoxynol-9 (see page 150). The addition of the spermicide is designed to kill spermatozoa in the immediate vicinity of a spilled condom and is not designed to replace the preferred combination of condoms and spermicidal foam, although it does add an extra small measure of protection.

Most reasons for condom failure stem from error in use such as inconsistent use of the method, vaginal penetration before the condom is applied, failure to unroll the condom for its entire length over the penis, not leaving sufficient space at the tip for the ejaculate, or not withdrawing the penis before it becomes flaccid so that semen spills in the vagina. Of course, failures can also occur from breakage during intercourse or, more rarely, from tearing of the condom while it is being unrolled and placed on the penis.

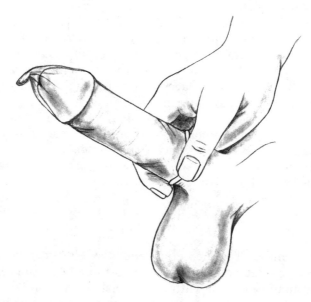

Figure 4-10. *Space should be left at the end of the condom to hold the ejaculate and help prevent rupture or spillage.*

Marketing. In spite of their many potential benefits, the use of condoms has been hampered by the widely held belief that they are a hindrance to sexual expression, intimacy, and pleasure. This belief is outmoded and overlooks modern improvements in condom design and sensitivity. It also ignores changes in the degree of sexual communication among modern couples. Condoms are an important contraceptive and the best protection against sexually transmitted diseases (STDs; see Chapter 7).

Studies have suggested that many couples in the United States reject condoms because of the historical association of "rubbers" with illicit sex. They also tend to overlook the contraceptive benefit because they only think of condoms as a disease preventive. Another hindrance to condom use is their considerable expense. But the most serious obstacle today are those local community standards that inhibit advertising or open display of condoms.

Experience in other countries has shown that condoms can be successfully used by a significant proportion of the population. In Japan, for example, it is estimated that 78% of couples are condom users, and Japan's birth rate is quite low. The use of condoms can be increased when distribution is extended beyond clinics and health agencies to community shops through aggressive social marketing. Innovative promotion and distribution approaches have been particularly successful in Bangladesh, China, Colombia, India, Jamaica, Kenya, Mexico, Sri Lanka, and Thailand.

VAGINAL SPERMICIDES

Historical references to vaginal spermicides are found in ancient texts. All sorts of imaginative chemical preparations have been described over time, including rock salt and alum, peppermint juice, cedar oil and gum, and sponges soaked with lemon juice. Most of these preparations were strongly acid or alkaline or had a high saline content that inactivated sperm. The first commercially produced spermicidal product—pessaries containing quinine sulfate—were developed in England during the 1880s. Foaming spermicidal tablets became available in Germany during the 1920s, and mercury compounds offering improved spermicidal effectiveness were introduced in the 1930s. Surface-active agents (surfactants) were developed in the 1950s. These chemicals, found to be less irritating to the penile and vaginal tissues than prior spermicidal products, are the principal active ingredients in modern spermicidal preparations.

Selection

Vaginal spermicides can be used alone or in combination with condoms or a diaphragm. They are made up of two components: (1) an inert material that disperses in the vagina to mechanically block the passage of sperm and that at the same time acts as a carrier for (2) a chemical spermicide that immobilizes and kills sperm before they can reach the uterus. Together, the inert material and the spermicidal chemical create a protective barrier when inserted into the vagina near the cervix.

Vaginal contraceptives are manufactured in many forms—jellies and creams, melting suppositories, foaming tablets, and aerosol foams. Most modern products rely on the spermicide nonoxynol-9. A notable exception is Neo-Sampoon, the Japanese foaming tablets that contain menfegol or TS-88. Both nonoxynol-9 and menfegol are surface-active agents that, on contact, coat and break down the surface of sperm cells. Menfegol has not at this time been approved by the Food and Drug Administration (FDA) for general use in the United States.

Advantages and disadvantages.   Vaginal spermicides offer the following advantages to users:

- Spermicides are the only female method of birth control that do not require medical intervention. They are readily available over the counter from commercial sources without prescription or the need for medical consultation.
- Spermicides are a simple, easily understood method of fertility control that is acceptable to some women who might not otherwise use family planning.
- They are apparently very safe, with no proven complications, although some users do report vaginal irritation, most frequently with the foaming suppositories.
- They can serve as a lubricant for intercourse, which may be beneficial to some couples.
- They are probably, to some degree, protective against sexually transmitted diseases.

Nevertheless, despite these advantages, certain intrinsic characteristics of spermicidal preparations have most likely contributed to their limited acceptance:

- Vaginal contraceptives have a generally higher failure rate than most other contraceptive methods.

- Foaming tablets and suppositories require waiting times of 3–10 minutes between insertion and intercourse to allow for adequate dispersal in the vagina.
- Spermicides must be applied immediately before each act of intercourse and remain effective for only a short time after insertion.
- Use of spermicides requires manipulation of the genitals, which may be offensive to some clients.
- Many couples consider spermicides "messy" and aesthetically unpleasant.
- The means of inserting the spermicide is sometimes awkward, and packaging can be bulky and obtrusive.

Contraindications. Contraindications to the use of spermicides are rare. Vaginal contraceptives should be avoided, however, if the woman or her partner is allergic to the ingredients or if high contraceptive effectiveness is essential. Spermicides may need to be temporarily avoided in the presence of any vaginal irritation.

Use

Client instruction. For effective use of vaginal spermicides, both timing and placement must be correct. Most important, the spermicide must be used each time intercourse occurs. If intercourse is repeated, another dose must be inserted into the vagina.

Spermicides are formulated with one of two types of base mediums or carriers. One type of base does not mix with semen, but rather acts as a barrier to semen diffusion. This type of spermicide is used with the diaphragm and includes brands such as Ortho and Ortho-Gynol creams and jellies and Koromex cream and jelly. The other type of spermicide base is miscible—it mixes with semen immediately so that the spermicidal agent can reach the spermatozoa quickly and destroy them. This type of spermicide is *not* used with a diaphragm but can be an effective adjunct to condom use or can be used alone with less effectiveness. This miscible type usually comes as a foam but sometimes as a cream and includes such brands as Conceptrol, Delfen, and Emko.

Melting contraceptive suppositories are inserted by hand deep into the vagina 15–20 minutes before intercourse (Figure 4-11). Suppositories are designed to melt at body temperature and release a spermicidal chemical. Vaginal foaming tablets usually consist of spermicide mixed with tartaric acid and bicarbonate of soda powder. This mixture effervesces in the presence of vaginal secretions 3–

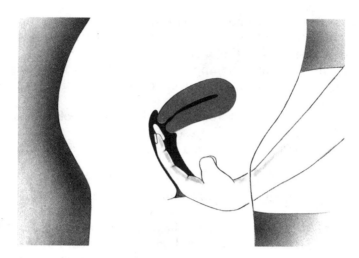

Figure 4-11. *Spermicidal vaginal suppositories.*

10 minutes after insertion, to generate a contraceptive foam. Melting suppositories and foaming tablets are conveniently small and easy to carry and use. Their effectiveness may be reduced, however, if they do not dissolve or effervesce completely—an unfortunately common occurrence. They can be a problem as well in warm humid climates since heat causes softening within the package. Placement of the packaged suppository or tablet under cold water for several minutes can usually harden the spermicide enough to allow handling.

Aerosol spermicidal foam, available in pressurized cans, is inserted deep into the vagina just prior to intercourse (Figure 4-12). A special applicator is used for insertion. Coital movements spread foam over the cervix. A major advantage of foam is that it disperses rapidly and evenly in the upper vagina and requires no waiting time between application and coitus. In contrast, vaginal foaming and melting tablets usually require 3–20 minutes for complete spermicide dispersal. Foam is the most effective and reliable of the vaginal spermicides used alone and is the most widely used. Like foaming and melting tablets, the effectiveness of the aerosol foam can be significantly increased if certain basic instructions are provided to the user:

- Several brands of foam are available in ready-to-use preloaded applicators. If the foam comes in a separate container, the

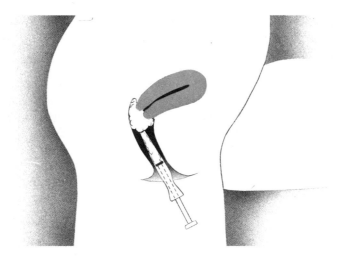

Figure 4-12.   *Spermicidal foam uses a special applicator.*

woman should be instructed to vigorously shake the can several times and then to fill the applicator to the designated
mark as directed on the package.
• The woman should insert the foam applicator as deep into the
  vagina as possible and withdraw it slightly, and then press the
  plunger to deposit the foam. The applicator should be removed carefully and washed for reuse later.
• If more than 30 minutes elapses before intercourse, another
  dose should be inserted and an additional full application
  used before each additional act of intercourse.

Side-effects.   The safety of vaginal contraceptives has generally
not been questioned, but adequate information on their long-term
effects is scarce. Concern has been increasing about localized skin
reactions in both sexual partners and also about possible systemic
effects. It has been recently discovered that nonoxynol-9 can be absorbed through the mucous membranes. Absorption through the vagina into the circulation could possibly harm the woman or harm
her infant if she is breastfeeding. Deleterious effects theoretically
could occur in men from ingestion of nonoxynol-9 if oral sex occurs
after insertion of the spermicide. Such effects have never been clinically demonstrated.
    Two preliminary studies have found an increased incidence of
congenital abnormalities in the offspring of women who used vagi-

nal spermicides near the time of conception. So far, these concerns are speculative but are now being researched. The U.S. FDA recently reapproved spermicides as safe drugs.

Effectiveness. Good data on the effectiveness of vaginal spermicides are deficient. Existing studies vary greatly in design, so comparisons of different spermicidal products are difficult. Interpretation of study results is complicated. A misleading negative impression can be obtained from some research because the failure of barrier methods is seldom due to failure of the product itself. It is more usually the result of inconsistent or incorrect use. On the other hand, the high effectiveness achieved in those clinical trials in which close follow-up is maintained and motivation is strongly reinforced is also misleading. Such studies do not present a true picture of the effectiveness of spermicidal preparations that are purchased over the counter and used without formal instructions.

The theoretical effectiveness of vaginal spermicides is estimated to be as high as 97% when used correctly. Use effectiveness, however, has been found to be much lower—about 78%. As mentioned earlier, though, vaginal spermicides can be very effective when used in combination with condoms.

Effectiveness varies considerably among the different types of spermicide. Aerosol foams are generally the most effective, probably because they disperse immediately. The effectiveness of foaming tablets and melting suppositories is lower because of their inherent inadequacies in creating a sufficient barrier. Furthermore, the waiting times necessary for spermicidal dispersal that vary from product to product are confusing to the user and aggravate low use effectiveness. Although spermicidal creams and jellies are recommended for use only with a diaphragm, their over-the-counter availability makes it possible for them to be used alone. Such improper use results in particularly low effectiveness.

The usefulness of vaginal spermicides could be improved by increasing the potency of the chemical spermicides themselves and by improving the ability of the inert carriers to (1) spread rapidly and evenly over the cervical opening and (2) hold the spermicide in the proper place for long periods of time. Research into improving vaginal spermicides has been sorely lacking, unfortunately; yet a reliably effective, convenient spermicide, if developed, could be an ideal contraceptive alternative.

FUTURE TRENDS AND
CONCLUSION

Public financing for research in and development of new barrier methods has been scanty. Likewise, little research has been undertaken by private companies because barrier methods are unlikely to provide a significant financial return. Nevertheless, some new products are currently being developed and tested. These include two types of contraceptive sponges; refined versions of the cervical cap, including a cap fit by customized casting; and other intravaginal devices designed to be longer-acting and/or disposable.

The two sponges are of particular interest. They are designed to provide an effective barrier that has less stringent requirements for time of insertion and removal. The Today sponge (formerly called Collatex) is a disposable polyurethane sponge containing approximately 1 g of nonoxynol-9. The sponge is inserted much like a diaphragm, up against the cervix. The sponge itself acts as a barrier while the spermicide, when in contact with vaginal secretions, disperses immediately across the cervical surface. It can be inserted long before intercourse, and the same sponge can be left in place and used for multiple acts of intercourse. Since the sponge comes in one universal size, no fitting is needed; it is intended to be sold over the counter and should be quite inexpensive.

In the testing that has been conducted so far, the contraceptive effectiveness rates for the Today sponge have been found to be between the highest rates achieved with the diaphragm and those achieved with the use of vaginal spermicides alone. The only identified contraindications to use of the Today sponge seem to be uterine prolapse and extremely lax pelvic musculature. Because the sponge is used repeatedly without removal, some users have complained that it develops unpleasant odors. This problem can be solved by replacing the sponge with a new one or by removal and washing. Apparently the sponge can be washed several times and still be effective, but enough washings will rinse out the spermicide. This sponge's unique characteristics may make it a particularly advantageous method for clients with irregular and unpredictable intercourse patterns, such as adolescents.

The collagen sponge differs from the Today sponge in two aspects: it is made of purified bovine (cow) collagen, not plastic; and it does not use any spermicide. Rather, the fibrous, mazelike collagen binds the ejaculate, trapping the sperm and preventing entrance into the cervix. On the basis of small field trials, effectiveness rates equal those of the Today sponge. But since the collagen sponge depends entirely on absorption of semen for its barrier effect, clinical testing on a larger scale will be required to prove that adequate effectiveness can be achieved without a spermicide.

The cervical cap is an old idea, but a new design may revive it as an effective barrier method. The cap differs from the diaphragm in that it fits *around* rather than in front of the cervix. One problem often cited in relation to traditional cervical caps is their inability to allow discharge of uterine and cervical secretions. A new cervical cap—the Contracap—is molded from an impression cast taken from each individual user. It has a valve "matrix" that permits secretions to pass through it while preventing sperm from entering. This custom-fitted cap could thus theoretically be left in place for weeks, even during menstruation. This intriguing idea is being investigated further.

Although large-scale clinical trials have not yet been conducted on any of these three methods, they offer hope for new contraceptive alternatives in the not-too-distant future. One or more of these alternative barrier methods could offer the unique combination of contraceptive effectiveness, convenience, accessibility, and safety that people are seeking.

Selected Readings

Anonymous: New contraceptive cap custom-made for cervix. Intercom: 2, May 1979

Anonymous: Collatex sponge: Condom equivalent for women? Contraceptive Technology Update 1(4): 49, July 1980

Balog J, Langhauser C, Rhine I: Recent trend in preference of contraceptive methods: Pills down, diaphragm on rise: A retrospective evaluation. Contraception 15(5): 553, May 1970

Bruce J, Schearer SB: Contraceptives and Common Sense: Conventional Methods Reconsidered. New York, Population Council, 1979, 125 pp

Chvapil M, Chvapil T, Jacobs S, et al: Laboratory and clinical testing of an intravaginal contraceptive collagen sponge. Contraception 15(6): 693, June 1977

Chvapil M, Droegemueller W, Owen JA, et al: Studies of nonoxynol-9. I. The effect on the vaginas of rabbits and rats. Fertility and Sterility 33(4): 445, April 1980

Coleman S and Piotrow PT: Spermicides—simplicity and safety are major assets. Population Reports H(5), September 1979

Connel EB: Cervical caps. Medical Aspects of Human Sexuality 12(11): 81, November 1978

Cutler JC, Aingh B, Carpenter U, et al: Vaginal contraceptives as prophylaxis against gonorrhea and other sexually transmissible diseases. Advances in Planned Parenthood 12(1): 45, 1977

Dalsimer IA, Piotrow PT, Dumm JJ: Condom—an old method meets a new social need. Population Reports H(1), December 1973

Dumm JJ, Piotrow PT, Dalsimer IA: The modern condom—a quality product for effective contraception. Population Reports H(2), November 1974

Edelman DA: Barrier contraception—an update. Advances in Planned Parenthood 14(4): 144, 1980

Edelman DA: Nonprescription vaginal contraception. International Journal of Gynecology and Obstetrics 18(5): 340, 1980

Edelman DA, Thompson S: Vaginal contraception—an update. Contraceptive Delivery Systems 3: 74, 1982

Felman YM: A plea for the condom, especially for teenagers. Journal of the American Medical Association 241(23): 2517, June 8, 1979

Gorline LL: Teaching successful use of the diaphragm. American Journal of Nursing 79: 1732, October 1979

Hatcher RA, Stewart GK, Stewart F, et al: Contraceptive Technology 1980–1981. New York, Irvington Publishers, 1980, 260 pp

Huggins G, Vessey M, Flavel R, et al: Vaginal spermicides and outcome of pregnancy: Findings in a large cohort study. Contraception 25(3): 219, March 1982

Jackson M, Berger GS, Keith LG: Vaginal Contraception. Boston, Hall, 1981, 255 pp

Jick H, Hannan MT, Stergachis A, et al: Vaginal spermicides and gonorrhea. Journal of the American Medical Association 248(13): 1619, October 1, 1982

Jick H, Walker AM, Rothman KJ, et al: Vaginal spermicides and congenital disorders. Journal of the American Medical Association 245(13): 1329, April 3, 1981

Kelaghan J, Rubin GL, Ory HW, et al: Barrier-method contraceptives and pelvic inflammatory disease. Journal of the American Medical Association 248(2): 184, July 9, 1982

Lane ME, Arceo R, Sobrero AJ: Successful use of the diaphragm and jelly by a young population: report of a clinical study. Family Planning Perspectives 8(2): 81, March/April 1976

Mills JL, Harley EE, Reed GF, et al: Are spermicides teratogenic? Journal of the American Medical Association 248(17): 2148, November 5, 1982

Oliva G, Cobble J: A reappraisal of the use and effectiveness of the diaphragm: An appropriate modern contraceptive. Advances in Planned Parenthood 14(1): 27, 1979

Richardson AC, Lyon JB: The effect of condom use on squamous cell cervical intraepithelial neoplasia. American Journal of Obstetrics and Gynecology 140(8): 909, August 15, 1981

Rothman KJ: Spermicide use and Down's syndrome. American Journal of Public Health 72(4): 399, April 1982

Shapiro S, Slone D, Heinonen OP, et al: Birth defects and vaginal spermicides. Journal of the American Medical Association 247(17): 2381, May 7, 1982

Sherris JD: Update on condoms—products, protection, promotion. Population Reports H(6), Baltimore, Johns Hopkins University, September/October 1982

Tatum HJ, Connell EB: Barrier contraception: A comprehensive overview. Fertility and Sterility 36(1): 1, July 1981

Tyrer LB, Bradshaw LE: Barrier methods. Clinics in Obstetrics and Gynecology 6(1): 39, April 1979

Vessey MP, Lawless M, Yeates D: Efficacy of different contraceptive methods. Lancet 1: 841, April 10, 1982

Williford JF: Barrier methods of contraception: Problems and prospects for the developing world. Draper Fund Report No. 6: 9, Summer 1978

Wortman J: The diaphragm and other intravaginal barriers: A review. Population Reports H(4), January 1976

Wright NH, Vessey MP, Kenward B, et al: Neoplasia and dysplasia of the cervix and contraception: A possible protective effect of the diaphragm. British Journal of Cancer 38(2): 273, August 1978

Zatuchni GI, Sobrero AJ, Speidel JJ, et al: Vaginal Contraception: New Developments. New York, Harper and Row, 1979, 389 pp

Uterine
Aspiration

5

A provider of health care to women will frequently find a need to perform uterine aspiration. Occasionally this will be necessary for the diagnosis of abnormal uterine function; most often it will be for termination of an unwanted pregnancy. Although not all health providers feel comfortable in personally performing abortions, there is no doubt that every provider will have to at least arrange for referral. For those practitioners choosing to deliver this essential health service, this chapter describes in detail the latest atraumatic techniques for safe, simple, and effective uterine aspiration. Emphasis is placed on those techniques that use flexible plastic cannulas (aspirating tubes).

Until the ideal contraceptive method is developed and used by all who need it, abortion will remain a necessary if unfortunate component of a family planning service. The experience of an unwanted pregnancy is often the beginning of consistent and conscientious contraceptive use. Seeing the client for an abortion is an excellent opportunity for contraceptive motivation. Furthermore, a family planning provider's own clients may return with an unwanted pregnancy caused by a failure of their chosen contraceptive method. The provider is therefore obligated to provide abortion as a back-up service.

Finally, some women will first be seen by a health provider because of complications from a septic incomplete abortion induced elsewhere. This will be particularly true when safe pregnancy termination services are not freely available. In many developing countries the majority of beds in the obstetrical wards are occupied by victims of septic incomplete abortion. Use of the atraumatic aspiration techniques described in this chapter for the treatment of these women can save many lives.

TERMINOLOGY

A number of terms have been used by researchers and practitioners to describe the technique of aspiration of the uterine cavity with flexible cannulas. This plethora of names has resulted from differing criteria for the procedure and from a desire to use euphemistic wording in situations where more traditional terminology would be misleading or offensive. The essential feature of flexible cannula uterine aspiration techniques is that the uterine cavity is efficiently evacuated *without forceful or excessive dilation of the cervix.* The appropriateness of one term or another to describe any particular procedure is dependent on the indications of the procedure—whether diagnostic or therapeutic—and the individual woman's physical condition and laboratory findings.

When pregnancy is a clinical consideration in uterine aspiration, semantic confusion results from differing ways to measure the length of gestation. The most useful method of dating the duration of pregnancy is calculating the interval from the first day of the woman's last menstrual period (LMP) to the time of examination. This method of dating, rather than from the estimated date of ovulation or from the date of the missed period, is used in this chapter to avoid confusion.

In this chapter we use three terms: *menstrual induction, endometrial biopsy,* and *suction curettage,* which are defined in Table 5-1. We concentrate on an aspiration procedure that does not require a reliable positive pregnancy test and is performed *after the 35th and up to the 50th* day since the last menstrual period. Although the phrase "menstrual regulation" is the more common term for flexible cannula uterine aspiration, it has most often been used to apply to procedures performed before *42 days LMP.* When aspiration is performed so early, before conventionally available pregnancy tests can reliably detect pregnancy, the proportion of unnecessary aspirations is higher than when the same technique is used slightly later. Thus we use the phrase "menstrual induction" to distinguish our gestational criteria of 35–50 days LMP. We recognize, however, that "menstrual regulation" has been acquiring increasing acceptance in describing this procedure.

Table 5-1.
Uterine Aspiration: Terms and Definitions.

Menstrual induction: aspiration of the uterus, not requiring a pregnancy test, performed 35–50 days LMP

Suction curettage: uterine aspiration for termination of pregnancy after 50 days LMP

Endometrial biopsy: uterine aspiration for solely diagnostic purposes

Treatment of incomplete abortion: aspiration to complete the removal of uterine contents that remain after incomplete spontaneous or induced abortion

Unfortunately, menstrual induction has been used by some researchers to refer to pregnancy termination through the use of medications called *prostaglandins.* "Menstrual extraction" has also been used by some authors to refer to flexible cannula uterine aspiration, but because of the varying gestational criteria used, the term is confusing.

The word that may seem the most direct—"abortion"—is heavy with unfortunate connotation and legal significance. The word is sometimes misleading when describing flexible cannula procedures, since in many of the clinic situations in which they have been used the preprocedural diagnosis of pregnancy has remained questionable.

Another therapeutic application of uterine aspiration techniques with significant public health implications is the treatment of *incomplete abortion.* Spontaneous abortions occur without outside intervention in 5%–10% of all pregnancies; occasionally the provider will see women in whom the spontaneous abortion was incomplete, with products of conception remaining in the uterus. Also, pregnancy termination sought from nonprofessional operators often results in incomplete evacuation and dangerous intrauterine sepsis. When a woman presents with acute hemorrhage, especially when combined with symptoms of infection, septic incomplete abortion should be assumed. The uterine aspiration techniques described here are well suited for the treatment of these cases.

Endometrial biopsy is the uterine aspiration technique used when the procedural indication is entirely diagnostic rather than therapeutic and pregnancy is not suspected regardless of the period of amenorrhea.

Since performing uterine aspiration late in the first trimester (after the seventh week LMP) is sometimes unavoidable, we briefly discuss aspiration by use of rigid cannulas and vacuum sources of more capacity, which we call *suction curettage*. Most of this chapter, however, is oriented to the flexible cannula technique that is easily learned by even nonphysician health providers.

CURRENT TECHNOLOGY

A woman faced with a delayed menstrual period and a possible unwanted pregnancy previously had only a few undesirable alternatives available. Fifteen to 20 years ago, this was true everywhere; in some places it is still true. A woman knew she had to wait several weeks before pregnancy could be confirmed and an abortion performed—somewhere, at some price, with questionable legal status. If she waited too long or did not decide to have an abortion until the pregnancy was well established, she could be by then in her second trimester of pregnancy. At best she could only hope for a complicated hospital-based saline abortion as an alternative to a dangerous illegal procedure.

Today this situation has significantly changed through the development of flexible plastic instruments of small diameter. A woman faced with a possible but unconfirmed and unwanted pregnancy can walk into a health clinic or doctor's office and, often in less than an hour, have a safe and complete uterine evacuation—with minimal pain, little physical trauma, and less threatening psychological pressure. This is the dramatic progress in health care that menstrual induction represents.

The safety and essential simplicity of menstrual induction is in vivid contrast to the agony of dangerous and haphazard techniques that result in septic abortion. Tragically, this still occurs by the thousands daily around the world. With the most basic plastic equipment and careful training, even nonphysician health personnel can provide a safe alternative.

Advantages

There are three distinct advantages of menstrual induction when compared with other abortion methods: it is physically and psychologically atraumatic, it can be performed very early in gestation, and it is technically relatively simple.

Atraumatic. As is described in detail here, the most obvious distinction of menstrual induction compared to other abortion methods is that it does not require forcible dilation of the cervix. With the use of cannulas of 6 mm in diameter or less and an atraumatic tenaculum, the reproductive organs are minimally affected by the procedure. Only removal of the uterine lining is accomplished; the internal os remains virtually undisturbed.

Early. Ample evidence has accumulated to show that early aspirations are *safer*, with fewer short- and long-term complications. Furthermore, since menstrual induction may be safely performed before a routine pregnancy test can be accurately used, the woman seeking this procedure need not necessarily face the *fact* of pregnancy—a psychological distinction of potential advantage or disadvantage considering the religious and social conflicts surrounding pregnancy termination.

Simple. Trained physician or nonphysician health providers can safely perform menstrual induction—a tremendous advantage wherever physicians are in short supply and the need for abortion services is high. Certified nurse-midwives or skilled nurses with special training are already effectively delivering menstrual induction as part of family planning services in some areas, relieving a significant burden from the gynecologist and general practitioner. When properly integrated into a total family and maternal health service, menstrual induction is practicable in remote field areas. Nonphysician delivery of menstrual induction can make a major contribution to world maternal health by replacing crude and hazardous abortion methods with a decidedly safer procedure.

HISTORY

Anthropological evidence indicates that induced abortion is as old as humans themselves—the oldest surgical procedure known. Methods of preventing birth, either before or after conception, were discussed in the earliest known medical writings, including Egyptian papyrii dating from 1850 to 1550 B.C. Regulations on abortion appear in the codes of all ancient civilizations including Sumer, Assyria, Bablylonia, and Persia. Although subject to numerous conditions and admonitions, abortion was approved and encouraged by

Plato and Aristotle. Abortion methods were also discussed in the early texts of China by Sun Ssu Mo in the 7th century A.D. and in the earliest Islamic medical texts of Rhazes in the 10th century A.D.

Religious Debates

The history of abortion is wrapped in the shrouds of complex moral and religious debates. The earliest Hindu scriptures, the Vedas (2000–80 B.C.), discussed induced abortion and termed it a serious sin. The Hindu scriptures set standards for the holiest of people however, and Hindu laws written for the common person provided conditions in which abortion would be permissible.

Early Islamic writings considered children to be gifts from God, making it a sin to induce abortion. But as recently as December 1964, high Islamic authorities declared it permissible to induce abortion before the embryo has assumed a "human shape." Most Moslem scholars now agree that abortion is permissible under varying conditions at up to 120 days of gestation.

Early Jews and Christians, whose small numbers demanded procreation to preserve their existence, viewed induced abortion as a major sin; yet again conditions have been described and continually expanded in which abortion is permissible in these religions. It is only since the mid-19th century that Roman Catholic doctrine has so strictly prohibited abortion. The French historian Devereux concluded that "abortion is an absolutely universal phenomenon."

Technological Development

The technique of menstrual induction dates from the development of methods for examining the interior of the uterus by curettage. This procedure has always been a basic part of gynecological practice that often requires examination of the endometrium and uterine contents. Medical records from Europe in the Middle Ages show that leeches were placed in the upper vagina to draw blood and "cleanse" the uterus—a procedure somewhat akin (at least in intent) to menstrual induction. In the 19th century, a few pioneering gynecologists sought to greatly simplify diagnostic curettage in order to make it a much safer and easier procedure. Queen Victoria's gynecologist, Sir James Young Simpson, of Edinburgh, used a narrow ivory tube, ¾ inch in diameter, and a syringe to put leeches onto the cervix. He also put holes into a catheter tube and attached the tube to an exhausting syringe to induce menstruation in cases of amenorrhea.

In 1924 two doctors in the United States first described successful diagnostic uterine curettage as an office procedure. In 1927 Bykov of the Soviet Union developed a crude vacuum aspirator by fitting a hollow cone-shaped tube over the end of a simple syringe. The syringe produced a negative suction of around 40 cm of mercury, causing menstruation within a few days. The whole procedure took less than 10 minutes. In this manner, Bykov prevented pregnancy in 25 women and thought that the procedure could be used once a month as a method of contraception.

Suction curettage by use of an electrically generated vacuum was developed in Hungary and in the United States in 1935. It was first used as a test for secretory endometrium in infertility cases. The electric vacuum technique was refined by Chinese physicians in 1958 and Soviet physicians in 1961. The breakthrough in the development of menstrual induction came in the late 1960s when Harvey Karman in California applied the new technology of flexible polyethylene tubing to the suction curettage concept. This design was further refined in the early 1970s. The first studies of this new atraumatic procedure with the plastic hand-operated vacuum syringe were published in 1971.

In all its variations, the most universal method of fertility control continues to be practiced all over the world. Although some women are benefiting from modern, simple, and inexpensive techniques of atraumatic uterine aspiration, too many others—in areas rich and poor, urban and rural—are still employing ancient methods of inducing abortion at great risk to their health and security. These methods include the violent uterine massage common in Southeast Asia, the herbal potions administered orally or vaginally in many parts of Africa, and the proverbial knitting needles still resorted to almost everywhere. Anyone who views the consequences of these desperate acts is strongly moved to make safe abortion techniques widely known.

FUNDAMENTALS

Anatomy

In order to understand the advantage and special applicability of the menstrual induction technique, it is first necessary to understand the features of uterine anatomy and physiology that permit the use of this procedure.

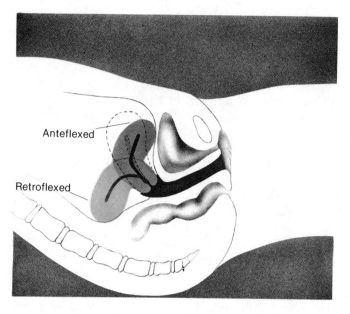

Figure 5-1. *Uterine flexion.*

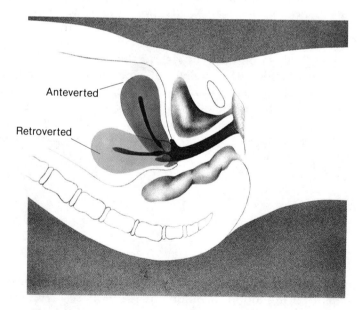

Figure 5-2. *Uterine version. An anteverted uterus is most common.*

166

The uterus is a pear-shaped organ composed primarily of involuntary muscle called *myometrium*. Its cavity is lined by a mucous membrane called the *endometrium*. The upper portion of the uterus is covered by *peritoneum*, which extends from the sides of the uterus to the pelvic walls, passing over the more fibrous cardinal ligaments. The uterus is situated between the urinary bladder and the rectosigmoid colon (see Figure 3-8); its precise position in the pelvis is, however, subject to much individual variation.

The position and contour of the uterus is dependent on many genetic, developmental, and pathological factors too involved to discuss briefly. Nevertheless, it is essential to the understanding of the techniques of uterine aspiration to recognize the many possible normal variations in uterine anatomy and to be able to identify them.

The uterus usually lies somewhat curved on its long axis (along its length). This is called *flexion*. When curved up toward the urinary bladder, the position of the uterus is called *anteflexion*. *Retroflexion* is the term used to describe a uterus that curves backward toward the rectosigmoid colon (Figure 5-1).

Version is another term used to describe uterine position. It describes the position of the whole uterine structure in relation to the long axis of the vagina. In most cases the uterus is found in the anteverted position, meaning that the long axis of the uterus is directed more upward (toward the abdominal wall) than the long axis of the vagina. Retroversion is a less common, but still quite normal, position. A retroverted uterus projects downward from the vaginal vault toward the sacrum (Figure 5-2).

The *size and configuration* of the uterus is mainly dependent on the parity of the woman, though again, genetic, developmental, and pathological factors cause individual differences. In a young girl before puberty, or in the mature woman who continues to have an infantile uterus, the cervix is the dominant portion of the organ—comprising about two-thirds of the length of the uterus. The corpus or uterine body comprises the other one-third (Figure 5-3). In the parous woman the ratio is reversed: the corpus accounts for about two-thirds of the total uterine length. The adult nulliparous uterus is in between—half cervix and half corpus. The parous uterus is also somewhat larger in its overall dimensions than the nulliparous uterus.

The appearance of the cervix is also changed with parity. In the nulliparous woman, the cervix appears essentially round to oval in shape, and the external os (opening or entrance) is distinctly round. The parous woman has a more slitlike os, with the overall shape of

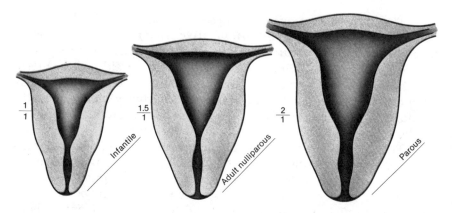

Figure 5-3.   *Comparative uterine sizes and proportions.*

the cervix somewhat more flattened (Figure 5-4). The cervix that has been previously dilated by childbirth is generally somewhat more elastic and is more easily manipulated and dilated.

The uterine cavity is somewhat triangular in shape, with the apex of the triangle at the internal os of the cervix. The base of the triangle (the farthest wall of the uterus) is the uterine *fundus*. The point at which the fallopian tubes join the uterine fundus is called the *cornual region*. Rarely, the uterine cavity is distorted by congenital malformations (see page 211). The cavity itself is flattened (Figure 5-5). Only when the cavity is distended by contents do the uterine walls significantly separate.

The mucous membrane lining the uterus, the endometrium, is a remarkable tissue that undergoes striking cyclic changes. The sur-

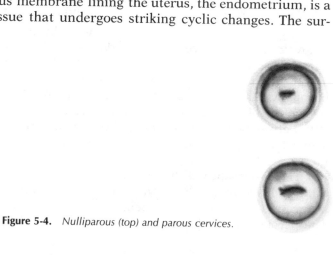

Figure 5-4.   *Nulliparous (top) and parous cervices.*

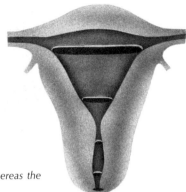

Figure 5-5. *The cervical canal is cylindrical, whereas the uterine cavity is triangular and flat.*

face of the endometrium consists of an undulating layer of columnar cells with deep glandular indentations. These glands become deeper and more complex in their shape as the menstrual cycle progresses. The supporting tissue just under the surface also undergoes complex cyclic changes, becoming increasingly filled with fluid and blood vessels. Most of the endometrium is shed with each menstrual period, with only the base of the glands remaining. Toward the end of menstruation, the changing hormonal stimuli cause these remnants to regenerate the complete endometrial lining in a very few days. The cycle then repeats: proliferation, secretion, maturation, and shedding—unless pregnancy interrupts the cycle (see Figure 2-2A).

Endometrial Biopsy

Disturbances in the regular pattern of menstrual cyclicity can be caused by conditions as diverse as psychological stress, infection, or pregnancy. Uterine aspiration is often an important tool in diagnosing the menstrual disruption. When samples of the uterine lining are aspirated for diagnosis in the nonpregnant uterus, the procedure is called *endometrial biopsy.* This is a useful application of the menstrual induction equipment but is distinct from the procedure done when pregnancy is suspected.

Microscopic examination of tissue obtained by endometrial biopsy can be of great help—and indeed in some circumstances is essential—in establishing the diagnosis of a variety of gynecological conditions (see Chapter 7). The tissue pattern of the aspirated material may disclose the hormonal state of the endometrium as well as show the presence of infection or other disease. Endometrial

(

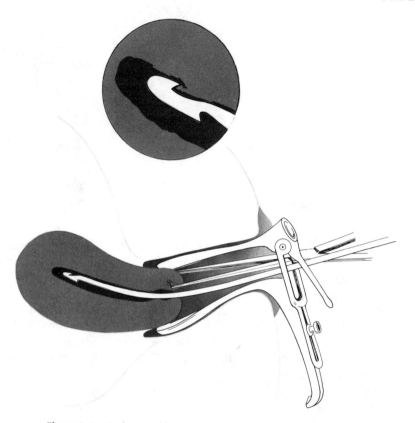

Figure 5-6.   *Endometrial biopsy is a valuable diagnostic procedure.*

biopsy is of value in the investigation of infertility problems, secondary amenorrhea, infectious disease, suspected endometrial cancer, and functional menstrual disturbances (Figure 5-6).

Infertility and inflammatory diseases of the pelvis are often interrelated. The relationship between tubal infection caused by gonorrhea and tubal occlusion is commonly recognized; however, the fact that a significant portion of infertility in some parts of the world results from pelvic tuberculosis is often forgotten or overlooked. The diagnosis of pelvic tuberculosis is often very difficult, particularly in the early stages. In these cases, material obtained by endometrial biopsy can be used in two very important diagnostic tests—a bacteriological examination for the bacillus and histological examination for the tissue pattern indicative of this condition.

The primary complaint of a woman with genital tuberculosis is usually infertility. In the United States, tuberculosis is a relatively rare cause of female infertility; in some other areas of the world, the incidence of tuberculosis is much higher and the disease is probably responsible for a great deal more infertility. Aspiration biopsy of the endometrium with special studies for tuberculosis is indicated in a woman complaining of infertility who has a positive skin test for tuberculosis.

Of course, much more diagnostic information can be obtained from the aspiration biopsy in the evaluation of infertility. If the procedure is done at a known time of the menstrual cycle (preferably in the immediate premenstrual phase or on the first day of menstruation), one can learn a great deal about the hormonal status of the patient. The degree of development of the uterine lining gives information about ovarian and pituitary function, and microscopic cellular changes will indicate whether ovulation has occurred and whether secretory changes have taken place in the endometrium. Endometrial biopsy frequently enables the clinician who knows the menstrual history of the patient to give a very close estimate of the date of ovulation and an assessment of the normalcy of the woman's hormonal status.

The aspiration biopsy may also be of use in the diagnosis and treatment of menopausal or postmenopausal bleeding problems and other menstrual irregularities. Sometimes the discovery of a clearly nonmalignant but pathological condition may be an important first step in the definitive diagnosis of the disease; it can be achieved through endometrial biopsy with simplicity and minimal effort. In cases of postmenopausal bleeding, however, negative findings from aspiration biopsy will not absolutely rule out an active adenocarcinoma (glandular cancer), and the patient will need to be followed closely.

Physiology of Early Pregnancy

In order to discuss the application of the uterine aspiration technique to the pregnant or possibly pregnant uterus, it is necessary to review the events and anatomical changes of early gestation. The process begins with ovulation, when the ovum is expelled from the follicle on the ovarian surface (Figure 5-7). Ovulation usually occurs around midcycle, about halfway between the beginning of one menstrual period and the next. Unfortunately, this timing is only approximate and cannot be relied on. Nevertheless, there are some physiological indications of ovulation that can be helpful. Ovulation is preceded in some women by a day or two of especially sticky mucoid vaginal discharge (mucorrhea). In some women, ovu-

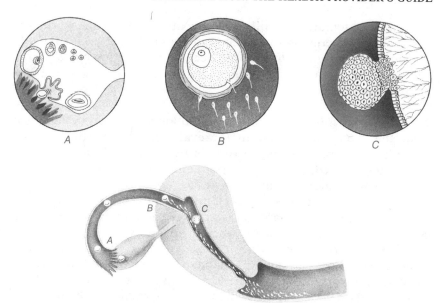

Figure 5-7. *Ovulation (A), fertilization (B), and implantation of the fertilized ovum in the endometrium (C).*

lation may be accompanied by a sharp lower abdominal pain of short duration called *mittelschmerz*.

After ovulation the egg travels down the fallopian tube, where fertilization may occur. Following coitus the spermatozoa find their way into the fallopian tubes by their own action and the muscular activity of the uterus. The egg is capable of being fertilized for only a matter of hours after ovulation, but the spermatozoa are capable of fertilizing for a considerable time, perhaps for as long as 5 days.

After fertilization the egg continues its 3-day journey down the fallopian tube and enters the uterine cavity. While the fertilized egg is traversing the tube, it undergoes several stages of cell division as it becomes a *blastocyst*. The blastocyst is a tiny fluid-filled ball of over 100 cells, only about 8 of which will contribute to fetal development, while the remainder will become components of the placenta.

Implantation occurs sometime after the blastocyst arrives in the uterine cavity, but the exact timing of this event is not known. Laboratory samples of early embryological material have shown that implantation can occur as early as the seventh postfertilization day and that the products of conception are well established on the uterine surface by the ninth postfertilization day. At the time of implantation the endometrium is in its secretory or progestational phase—the latter part of the menstrual cycle.

This receptivity of the endometrium is the result of the secretion of progesterone from the ovary. The ovarian follicle, which expelled the ovum and prior to ovulation had been producing estrogen, undergoes a striking change after ovulation. In its changed state the follicle is called the *corpus luteum* (yellow body). It begins the secretion of progesterone in addition to its continued secretion of estrogen. The progesterone secretion continues for 12–14 days, and it induces and maintains the receptive state of the endometrium. If fertilization and implantation does *not* occur, the progesterone secretion diminishes and ultimately ceases. Menstruation follows and a new cycle begins.

When fertilization *does* occur, however, a different chain of events takes place. The *trophoblast* (those cells of the blastocyst destined to become the placenta) begins the secretion of yet another hormonal substance, human chorionic gonadotropin (HCG), which stimulates the function of the corpus luteum and extends the secretory or progestational phase of the endometrium. The maintenance of the receptive state of the uterus is dependent on the ovarian secretion of progesterone for at least 4 weeks after ovulation. After that time, the trophoblast itself is able to secrete the necessary progesterone and the corpus luteum is no longer necessary to the continuation of pregnancy.

Meanwhile the trophoblast continues to secrete HCG in increasing quantities. Even before the time of the missed period, very minute amounts of HCG can be detected in the blood when special methods such as the beta subunit test are used. This provides an effective pregnancy test that can be performed very early in gestation. These tests are quite expensive, however, and not widely available. Secretion of HCG increases sufficiently by 42 days LMP (when the menstrual period is 2 weeks late) so that routine urine pregnancy tests will be accurate by that date.

The endometrium in which the egg is embedding is now called the *decidua*. It combines with the trophoblast to form the placenta. At the 12th day after fertilization—about the time when menstruation would have occurred—the ovum measures only about 1 mm across. The earliest beginnings of the amniotic sac are apparent, and within it is the embryonic disk—the small precursor of the embryo that is already differentiated from the majority of the cell mass. The most prominent feature of the fertilized egg at the time of the missed period is the trophoblast. It has separated into two layers

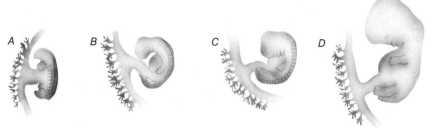

Figure 5-8. *Embyonic development: (A) 28 days, (B) 35 days, (C) 42 days, (D) 50 days LMP.*

and has formed fingerlike projections called *villi*. Those villi that are in contact with the decidua anchor firmly into the uterine lining. From a barely visible collection of cells at 28 days LMP, therefore, the placenta grows dramatically to a not inconsiderable volume of 10 ml or more at 50 days LMP and grows at an even faster rate in subsequent weeks (Figure 5-8).

Until 35 days LMP, all the products of conception together are generally referred to as the *blastocyst*. From about the 35th day on, the placenta is recognized as a distinct entity. The embryonic disk is by this time sufficiently differentiated and developed to be called an *embryo*. The embryonic phase persists for about 5 weeks, until 70 days LMP. This is an important time in gestation, for before this time the embryo has no recognizable human organ systems. By the

		Table 5-2.			
		Stages of Gestational Growth.			
Weeks of Gestation	**Days LMP**	**Diameter of Uterine Fundus**	**Depth of Uterine Sounding**	**Status of Development**	**Size**
4	28	6 cm	7 cm	Blastocyst	1 mm
5	35	6 cm	7 cm	Embryo	<1 mm
				(Amniotic sac 1 cm)	
6	42	6 cm	7–8 cm	Embryo	4–5 mm
7	49	7 cm	8 cm	Embryo	10 mm
8	56	8 cm	9 cm	Embryo	22–24 mm
10	70	10 cm	11 cm	Embryo–fetus	4 cm
12	84	11 cm	12+ cm	Fetus	7–9 cm

70th day LMP, the organ systems are defined and further development consists only of growth and maturation of these systems. After 70 days LMP, the organism is called a *fetus*. These different names for the products of conception are somewhat arbitrary and imprecise but do tend to reflect the dramatic changes that take place in the early weeks of pregnancy. Relative sizes and other dimensions at each of these stages is shown in Table 5-2. Uterine size and consistency during subsequent stages of pregnancy is described on page 193.

A thorough familiarity with these aspects of anatomy and physiology of the female reproductive system will greatly aid in understanding the applications of uterine aspiration in both pregnant and nonpregnant women and is essential to proper aspiration technique.

Concepts of Abortion

Delayed menstruation and slight changes in uterine size and texture do not necessarily prove that the woman is pregnant. If the possible pregnancy is unwanted or if it would be dangerous to the woman to have the pregnancy continue, uterine aspiration to terminate the suspected pregnancy should be considered.

The increased size, greater softness, and larger volume of contents of the pregnant uterus require greater care and caution when aspirating than when performing endometrial biopsy on a nonpregnant organ. As pregnancy progresses beyond the first few weeks, the diagnosis becomes more certain, but intervention can carry significant hazards, especially later in pregnancy, requiring procedures carefully selected as being appropriate to the situation.

The stages of pregnancy at which intervention is possible are primarily defined by social and legal constraints rather than by medical indications. In certain societies and jurisdictions abortion may be inappropriate at any stage of pregnancy—diagnosed or suspect. In other areas of the world restrictions do not apply.

The spectrum of alternative abortion methods according to gestational age is shown in Figure 5-9. In the second trimester of pregnancy (13–26 weeks LMP), abortion carries an increasingly greater risk than it does in the first trimester (up to 12 weeks LMP). In the second trimester the fetus and placenta have advanced in size and development. Operators with special training can evacuate the uterus with dilation and vacuum aspiration at 12–16 weeks LMP, or even beyond (dilation and evacuation, D&E), but the procedure is

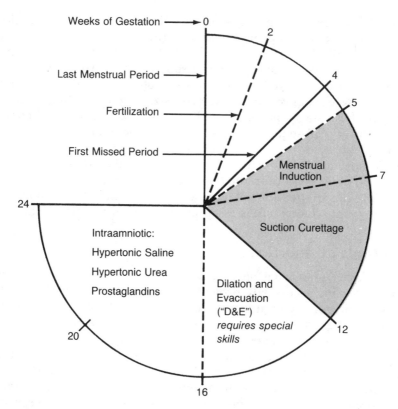

Figure 5-9. *Spectrum of abortion alternatives by weeks of gestation. Techniques discussed in this chapter are indicated by shading.*

more complex and requires a high degree of skill to avoid the usual hazards of midtrimester abortion.

Later in the second trimester, pregnancy terminations can also be performed by injecting hypertonic solutions (either sodium chloride or urea) or prostaglandins directly into the amniotic sac with a long needle (amniocentesis). This will usually initiate labor-like contractions within a few hours after the injection. Hypertonic saline is a highly toxic solution, and accidental placement of the saline into a blood vessel can be very dangerous. Before 16 weeks LMP the amniotic sac is very hard to find with the needle, making this method impractical until after the 16th week. This procedure obviously has a tremendous psychological impact on the patient—

she is in a hospital, she actually undergoes laborlike contractions, and a recognizable fetus is expelled. Unless saline induction is performed with the highest standards of sensitivity and care, it has the potential for long-term traumatic effects. Nevertheless, many women must still undergo saline abortions because legal, social, or psychological problems have delayed their decision to abort until the second trimester.

All second-trimester methods are often augmented by insertion of laminaria tents in the cervix for gentle dilation and by the intravenous infusion of oxytocin to induce uterine contractions. It is clear that in expert hands abortion in the second trimester can be performed with an acceptable degree of safety; however, in most instances it remains decidedly less desirable on psychological and medical grounds than first trimester abortion.

Before modern equipment was available, first-trimester abortion was performed by cervical dilation and uterine curettage (D&C) usually before the beginning of the 13th week from the LMP. This procedure requires forcible dilation of the cervix with metal dilators. The products of conception are removed by scraping the uterine wall with the ovum forceps and a metal curette. Because of the inherent dangers of metal instrumentation, an alternative for this procedure has been sought with less dilation and trauma.

The abortion method in widest use today uses gentle cervical dilation followed by suction curettage of the uterine contents by electric pump, using either flexible or rigid cannulas. This procedure is applicable any time after the establishment of the diagnosis of pregnancy but is usually performed after the 7th week and before the 13th week LMP. Impressive safety and effectiveness records have been achieved with this method, but it requires a better-equiped clinic than does menstrual induction and ready availability of emergency drugs and procedures (see page 204).

Menstrual induction occupies a special place in this spectrum of abortion alternatives. It is appropriate when menstruation has been delayed by only a week or more and can be used until such time as the uterine growth has become obvious (50 days LMP). It requires little, if any, cervical dilation and can be performed with a flexible plastic cannula of small diameter. A vacuum source of minimal capacity can be used, requiring no heat or electricity for power. A review of other abortion alternatives makes clear the advantages of this method that can be performed early, with little trauma, and with simplicity and speed.

EQUIPMENT AND FACILITIES

Aspiration Equipment

The cannula. The simplest equipment for modern atraumatic uterine aspiration is the flexible plastic cannula and aspiration syringe developed and refined during the 1970s. The cannula (often called the *Karman cannula*) is a flexible polyethylene tube of narrow diameter with a rounded tip. The cannula usually can be inserted into the uterus without other cervical dilation. The uterine contents are withdrawn through two lateral triangular-shaped openings located on opposite sides of the tip of the cannula. This tip will freely bend without blocking its openings. The tube is designed to fold when hitting the uterine fundus, preventing perforation (see Figure 5-20, inset).

An advantage of the plastic cannula over metal instruments is that its transparency enables the operator to watch the cannula for endometrial tissue, products of conception, or the air bubbles that signal that the procedure is completed. This cannula can also be used as a uterine sound. Some manufacturers embed a colored strip on the tube at a measured distance from the tip in order to mark uterine depth when inserting the cannula. The cannula's flexibility permits sounding with minimal danger of perforation. Another unique feature of the flexible cannula is that the cut of each opening at the tip acts as a curette while the suction draws on the uterine wall. This one flexible instrument thus combines the functions of dilation, sounding, aspiration, and curettage.

The vacuum source. The flexible cannula can be used with different sources of vacuum for aspiration. The simplest and most commonly used vacuum source is the plastic reusable 50-ml gynecological syringe (Figure 5-10). A vacuum of approximately 60 cm Hg is achieved by closing the pinch valve of the connecting adaptor and then withdrawing the rubber-tipped plunger until its locking handles are engaged. Held and operated by hand, the syringe maintains a vacuum adequate for uterine aspiration wihtout the use of electricity, manual pumping, or heat. Alternatively, vacuum pumps that operate by foot or electricity can also be used with the flexible cannula.

Gestational age is usually the determining factor in choosing a vacuum source. The gynecological syringe will generally be used for menstrual induction, and for pregnancies of most advanced gesta-

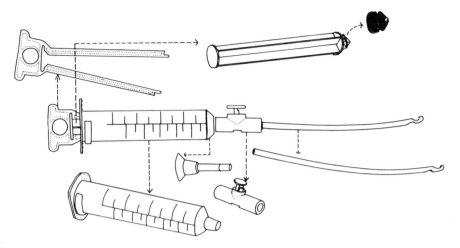

Figure 5-10. *Parts of the menstrual induction syringe.*

tion that are aspirated by suction curettage, electric suction machines will be used. These vacuum aspirators have large capacities and are needed for pregnancies of greater volume. Electric suction machines are connected to either flexible or rigid cannula by flexible plastic tubing and special connectors of larger diameter than used with the syringe.

Other factors besides gestational age may influence the suitability of a particular vacuum source. These factors include the preference of the provider, the cost and availability of the equipment and its maintenance, and the number of procedures being performed in the facility per day. Simple vacuum sources such as the gynecological syringe require little technical maintenance, are easy to use, and are dependable if used for *early* aspirations. Particularly busy clinics may find that electric suction machines are more appropriate even for menstrual induction procedures. Even if most of a clinic's procedures are menstrual inductions, it is advantageous to have vacuum sources of larger capacity on hand in case of inadvertent initiation of aspiration in a pregnancy too advanced for the syringe.

Cleaning and testing. The syringe is easily cleaned after each use by washing with soap or detergent and rinsing carefully. *The syringe should not be autoclaved:* this is unnecessary and shortens the syringe's useful life span. The plunger must be dried and lubricated with a silicone grease before storing. If silicone grease is not avail-

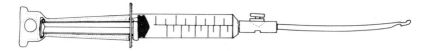

Figure 5-11. *The charged syringe, with pinch valve closed and plunger withdrawn.*

able, a thick solution of green soap, glycerol, or even water-soluble lubricating jelly may be used, but such materials should be applied only immediately prior to use, and not before storing.

In ordinary use and with careful maintenance, the syringe should last for 50 or more procedures. Nevertheless, before each use it should be tested to determine whether it can hold an adequate vacuum. By closing the pinch valve, withdrawing the plunger, and engaging the locking handles, the syringe is "charged" and set aside (Figure 5-11). After 2 minutes, the retracting lock is released, but not the pinch valve. If the plunger returns to within 3 mm or less of the valved end of the syringe barrel, the instrument's vacuum is adequate. If it fails this test, the plunger should be relubricated and the seal around the pinch valve checked. All syringes will eventually wear out, and when these simple remedies do not restore adequate performance, the syringe must be discarded.

Sterilization. The cannulas are initially supplied sterile. When they are reused they must be cleaned, carefully inspected, and rendered free of pathogens prior to another use. Gas sterilization (with ethylene oxide) is a safe and effective method but is not widely available. Other methods include soaking in a fresh aqueous solution of benzalkonium chloride (1:750) for 24 hours, or an aqueous iodine solution (1:2500) for 2 hours. Caution must be taken to ensure total immersion of all plastic surfaces. Prolonged exposure to iodine may make cannulas excessively rigid and brittle.

Supplies

In addition to the aspiration equipment, there are other supplies that are essential and some that are highly desirable. The basic uterine aspiration equipment includes a speculum, tenaculum, sponge forceps, sterile cotton balls, needle and syringe for paracervical block, and a small container for the antiseptic (Figure 5-12).

A small supply of emergency drugs should be available. This includes: an infusion set, along with the intravenous fluids used in an emergency such as Ringer's lactate; atropine sulfate for the occa-

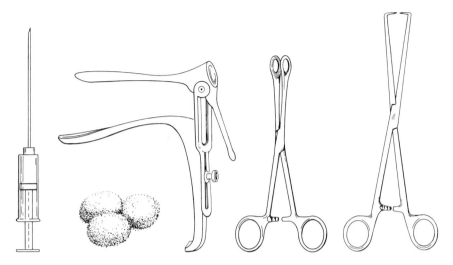

Figure 5-12. *Basic supplies for menstrual induction.*

sional patient who may have a vasovagal reaction (low blood pressure with a slow pulse); an ergot prepartion such as methylergonovine to induce uterine contractions; and syringes and needles suitable for either intravenous or intramuscular injection.

Facilities

The uterine aspiration clinic should have enough space to allow for patient counseling, examination, treatment, postprocedure rest, and record-keeping. If the clinic is a busy one, these functions require separate rooms. The counseling room must be quiet and private so that the woman can freely discuss her condition. The treatment room must be clean and well lighted, with a private area where the patient can undress. The examination table must be fitted with foot-stirrups or leg supports comfortable enough to allow the patient to remain in the lithotomy position for up to 15 minutes. A stool for the operator is also necessary, as is a table for the sterile instruments. The clinic should also have a comfortable bed or cot in a quiet location on which the patient can rest after the procedure if necessary.

An emergency medical facility should be adjacent or nearby the clinic for the treatment of any patient who might experience serious difficulty during or after the uterine aspiration procedure. Such a facility should have an operating room capable of providing conventional dilation and curettage or abdominal surgery and should be capable of providing adequate anesthesia. Emergency drugs and resuscitation equipment must also be available. Procedures for referral to this emergency facility should be worked out in advance, detailing how the patient in need can be transferred for immediate care.

If the emergency facility to be used for referral of special cases is relatively remote, or if the emergency facility is particularly busy, it is desirable to have available in the clinic an alternative source of vacuum of greater capacity than the menstrual induction syringe. Provided the clinic has a physician trained in the use of this equipment, complicated emergency referrals can be avoided if these larger vacuum sources are available.

PROCEDURE

The uterine aspiration procedure consists of several steps essential for safety and effectiveness. The client should first be counseled about her condition and the alternatives open to her. If she decides on uterine aspiration, a medical history should be taken, physical examination conducted, and laboratory tests performed if necessary. The procedural technique should then be carefully adapted to the woman's individual needs, follow-up instruction given, and contraceptive counseling provided. Each of these steps is discussed in detail in this section.

Counseling Considerations

Counseling is an integral part of any service offering early abortion. It serves to ensure the safety, humaneness, and dignity of the procedure and can greatly help to protect the woman at a time when she is vulnerable to damaging emotional and psychological influences.

Menstrual induction, like any abortion procedure, is not simply a "medical" experience. From the moment that the woman observes that her menstrual period is late until several months after the aspiration procedure, the experience of a possible unwanted pregnancy may have psychological and emotional effects on the woman. In this context, counseling has been called "preventive mental health."

In essence, counseling means that prior to performing an aspiration procedure, a trained staff member has individually talked with the patient at sufficient length about how she perceives her situation. The counselor assesses the reality of her perception, and presents the alternatives that may be solutions to her problem. But effective and quality counseling goes much further than this: it assists the patient in the implementation of her decision and provides her with education, motivation, and resources for contraception and other needs following the procedure. Ideally, counseling should involve the woman's sexual partner as well. This provides a rare opportunity for family planning contact with the male. In addition, his active support of the woman's decision can be a critical factor in the patient's emotional health.

The decision.   Puberty, pregnancy, and menopause have been described as the three biologically determined maturational crises in women. A request for abortion—regardless of whether pregnancy has been definitively diagnosed—indicates that for one reason or another, the woman must seek help in handling the crisis of pregnancy. The counselor's first job is to determine the extent of the problem and the reasons for it.

The counseling session should begin by exploring the patient's feelings about her possible pregnancy. She should be encouraged to talk about her own sexuality and her future fertility plans. Her fears and expectations about contraception should also be explored, and the counselor should begin even at this early stage to think about the appropriateness of the various contraceptive alternatives for the patient being interviewed.

The counselor must be especially careful to be entirely nonjudgmental in communication with the patient; it is critical that the woman undertake the procedure without influence from others. It is also important that the counselor be aware of the different backgrounds among the women that will be seen. Women of different ethnic, religious, and socioeconomic backgrounds require a counselor with the flexibility and understanding to adapt the counseling methods accordingly. Counselors must also be fully aware of their own feelings and assumptions about abortion, contraception, and sexuality.

The counseling session should include an explanation of the aspiration procedure—its advantages and disadvantages, its benefits and risks. The procedure should be described completely in language that the patient will easily understand, avoiding excessively detailed descriptions that may be unnecessarily frightening. The counselor can greatly relieve patient anxiety by anticipating the woman's fears and discussing them openly. Patience and sensitivity are important when explaining the procedure; many patients, even those who are supposedly well educated, are very poorly informed about their reproductive anatomy and physiology. It is imperative that the patient have a clear idea of what uterine aspiration means and involves both physically and emotionally before she agrees to the procedure.

Most, if not all, patients who seek abortion feel some degree of ambivalence about pregnancy. "Ambivalence" means that the patient is experiencing forces in two directions at the same time—both in favor and against continuation of the possible pregnancy. For many, this ambivalence may be only subtle and vague, since they have very strong motivation in one direction or the other. But for other patients the forces in *both* directions may be strong, resulting in emotional conflict. Such patients may need lengthy interviews and may find it very difficult to resolve their conflict.

Sometimes because of high degrees of ambivalence, sometimes out of fear of complications or discomfort, or sometimes because of a personality or character trait that makes decisions difficult, it may be very difficult to lead the patient toward a decision about her possible pregnancy. It is extremely important that the counselor refrain from losing patience or becoming judgmental by directing the patient to a conclusion. It is sometimes necessary, however, to be firm and controlling when the counseling process has been completed, and the patient must be told that her decision is required. When the patient is unable to decide, it must be interpreted as a decision against interference—a decision *against* abortion.

The counselor will see women with very different levels of family planning knowledge and emotional health. Some patients will be sophisticated and motivated family planners. Others will be secure, stable, and well-educated women who are not using contraception because of ambivalent feelings about pregnancy and sexuality. Many of the patients will be women who have not had access to family planning information or contraceptive services.

The younger patients are likely to be confronting their sexuality and the possibility of pregnancy for the first time. Sadly, many of these women with unwanted pregnancies will delay their decision to seek professional help. This delay can have serious consequences for the woman's health, since the complexity and risks of abortion increase in the second trimester. There are many causes of delay in seeking help: personal or partner ambivalence, family or religious pressures, or even a previous history of irregular menstruation.

Not the least prevalent reason for delay is the woman's perception of resistance or insensitivity among health care providers. The worst consequence of such provider attitudes is the woman carrying an unwanted pregnancy to term. Not only is this psychologically damaging to mother and child, it is also physically threatening to the mother: abortion by modern techniques is much safer than pregnancy. The provision of proper counseling services by the clinic can overcome the fears that cause delay. An active outreach program can encourage earlier clinical contact to prevent dangerous delays in decision-making.

Some patients may be chronic noncontraceptors with multiple previous abortions or contraceptive failures, whereas a few women will appear with multiple psychological and emotional problems in need of professional therapy. During the counseling process, certain of these patients will show a variety of symptoms of personality disorganization or frank mental illness. It must be remembered that a woman seeking uterine aspiration is a person in crisis; the stress may be sufficient to tear down defense mechanisms that have until now allowed a person with emotional problems to function adequately. The counselor must be prepared to recognize such patients and should be able to refer these women for proper psychiatric care. On the other hand, many normal women show strain from such a difficult crisis. Distinction between these two patient types requires sensitivity, experience, and concentration.

Those women seeking menstrual induction who are generally regarded to be in need of psychiatric referral are those with a history of psychosis or mental impairment; those who exhibit clinical depression, guilt, or hysterics; and those with evident suicidal tendencies. For a truly "therapeutic" intervention, these women require careful and expert psychiatric treatment before and after the procedure.

The support.   Once the patient has made a fully informed decision to undergo menstrual induction, the skillful counselor will help her with any necessary paperwork and will accompany her into the examination and treatment rooms. Throughout the process the counselor should give the woman information, instructions, emotional support, and even diversion in order to make the procedure easier for both the patient and the operator. The most important psychological consideration that the counselor and the operator can keep in mind is that the patient has rarely if ever been in this situation before, although *they* may be working with it every day. The counselor and the operator must never lose sight of this first-

time immediacy and apprehension in almost every one of their
patients.

The patient can be expected to be at least a little bit frightened,
since most patients have heard some terrible stories about abortion
experiences. The presence during the procedure of the same counselor who helped the patient sort out her feelings is clearly beneficial.
The counselor is able to give the woman the necessary instructions,
such as where to remove and store her clothes, when and where to
empty her bladder, and how to assume the proper position on the
treatment table. After the procedure has begun, the counselor can
lean down and talk intimately with the patient, reassuring her
about the sensations she is experiencing. This helps the patient to
anticipate discomfort without imparting fear of pain.

The supportive counselor contributes greatly to the ease with
which the aspiration procedure can be done, and many operators,
learning to rely on the skills of a counselor with whom they have
worked successfully before, begin to use less and less analgesia and
anesthesia for the procedure. Effective supportive counseling makes
these medications less important, resulting in faster postprocedure
recovery and release from the clinic, and probably in greater procedure safety as well.

During the procedure, the counselor informs the patient on a
step-by-step basis what the operation is about and why: explaining
the insertion of the speculum, the grasp of the tenaculum, the injection of the anesthetic, the insertion of the cannulas, the application of vacuum, and the possible cramping. If an intrauterine device (IUD) is elected as the postprocedure contraceptive method,
the counselor continues her supportive commentary during the
insertion.

Immediately after the procedure, while the patient is resting
and waiting for release, the counselor gives directions for follow-up
care and contraceptive practice. Special care must be taken at this
time to be absolutely certain that the patient fully understands the
postprocedure instructions. This period of time may provide a great
opportunity for family planning motivation; however, it is not likely
that the patient will be highly retentive of information. It is usually
advisable where appropriate to reinforce all the verbal instructions
with written ones.

The follow-up. The counselor shares with the operator the
responsibility of making sure that the patient keeps her return ap-
pointment for follow-up medical care and continuing contraceptive

support. Such a return is dependent on the patient perceiving the follow-up visit as valuable to herself and those who care about her. When the operator has delegated much of the patient contact to the skilled counselor, it becomes the counselor's responsibility to sincerely communicate to the patient that *both* members of the health service team really do care about her and will appreciate her return.

The return visit must include an exchange of ideas between the counselor and the patient. Again the patient should be encouraged to ventilate her feelings about her crisis, how she resolved it, and how she interprets the experience of the procedure. The patient's experience with her new method of contraception should also be discussed, and the counselor should reinforce prior instructions. Any new problems that may have developed because of the procedure, the method of contraception, or other aspects of the woman's sexuality, should be openly explored. This is often an opportune time to talk about the long-term advantages of child spacing and to reinforce motivation for family planning.

Choice of Procedure

Because of the rapid increase in the volume of uterine contents after the sixth week since the last menstrual period, and because of the increased dimension of the products of conception, the use of the menstrual induction technique is usually limited to those patients with a history of less than 50 days of amenorrhea. Very skilled and experienced practitioners may be able to extend the use of menstrual induction slightly beyond 50 days, but in the hands of less skilled or inexperienced practitioners, it is prudent to limit its use to even a few days less than 50 days LMP until the operator has acquired some experience. Pregnancies more advanced than 50 days LMP require cannulas of larger bore, more definitive cervical dilation, and vacuum sources of greater capacity (see page 204). Both provider and patient should always remember that the earlier the aspiration procedure is performed, the safer it will be.

Pregnancy tests. The technology for determining whether a woman is pregnant by chemical means is rapidly changing, leading to ever more sensitive tests. Nevertheless, pregnancy tests are only an adjunct to, not a requirement for, uterine aspiration. If the operator has a high degree of suspicion that the woman is pregnant and is at least at 42 days LMP, a pregnancy test is not necessary. On the other hand, it is desirable to minimize the performance of unnecessary aspiration procedures, so that if there is doubt in the operator's mind, or if it is necessary to perform uterine aspiration before 42 days LMP, a pregnancy test is useful.

Urine pregnancy tests are relatively inexpensive and easy to use and provide quick results. They are very reliable after 42 days LMP—the optimum time period for menstrual induction. A new group of "ultrasensitive" urine tests are reliable even earlier. They should be useful when they become more widely available and less expensive. The blood tests that look for human chorionic gonadotropin (HCG)—a key hormone found in the maternal circulation—are perhaps the most accurate in the critical period between 35 and 42 days. Blood HCG tests are much more expensive and not as widely available, however, and in the case of the beta subunit test, require sophisticated laboratory technique. The blood tests can be useful to providers with access to them when the physical findings are confusing, but their availability is by no means a requirement for a provider of uterine aspiration.

Since all urine pregnancy tests require some interpretation by the clinician, it is highly desirable to have the same well-trained person read all the test results at a single facility. This is especially true if the provider uses pregnancy tests only occasionally. Regardless of the type of test chosen, it is also important to store the test materials properly. The recommended storage conditions will be marked on the packaging.

Laboratory Studies

When a woman contacts a health provider for a family planning service, a special opportunity is offered for provision of other basic health services. Laboratory tests performed for women seeking menstrual induction must be kept in this perspective. No laboratory determinations are absolutely necessary, but several are desirable in varying degrees depending on the ability of the health care facility to deliver therapeutic services for those diseases that are disclosed by these tests.

Hematocrit or hemoglobin determination.   These blood tests will detect milder forms of anemia, and the provision of iron therapy to women so afflicted will have a positive effect on maternal health. Severe anemia is usually evident on physical examination without the need for a laboratory test. Severe anemia is not necessarily a contraindication to uterine aspiration, but may require in-patient rather than outpatient handling of the procedure. In any case, if the 50 days LMP time limit is strictly followed, total blood loss from this procedure will rarely exceed 30 ml, making these blood tests helpful but not mandatory.

Rh determination.   The Rhesus blood type should be determined for each patient undergoing uterine aspiration. Those patients who are Rhesus-negative and who have a pregnancy terminated should receive a prophylactic dose of Rh immunoglobulin.

The earliest time in pregnancy when Rhesus sensitization can occur is not known. The amount of embryonic blood prior to 50 days LMP is very small, however, and the fraction available for possible entry into maternal circulation and subsequent provocation of antibody formation is minute. Consequently, when menstrual induction is performed within 50 days LMP, the dose of immunoglobulin needed to be effective is very small.

Gonorrhea culture.   Any pelvic examination provides the opportunity for testing for gonorrhea. When facilities are available to culture gonococci, a smear of the cervical secretions and vaginal discharge (if any) should be taken and appropriate antibiotics made available if the test is positive. A positive culture need not preclude uterine aspiration, but *serious* pelvic infection of any kind may be a contraindication to an outpatient procedure.

Urinalysis.   Urinalysis is not a requisite test before menstrual induction but is clearly a desirable health care measure if resources for its provision and any subsequent therapy are available.

Papanicolaou smears.   An important health screening tool that is easily used with women seeking menstrual induction is the Papanicolaou smear test for the detection of cervical cancer. If facilities for interpretation of the smears are not available, however, or if therapeutic facilities to treat positive or suspicious results are not accessible as is true in many developing countries, obtaining these smears may be futile.

Patient History

Certain important elements of medical history should be gathered on all patients considered for menstrual induction procedures. The operator must be aware of the patient's previous operations (such as cesarean section), any serious illnesses that could interfere with the procedure (epilepsy, severe asthma, congestive heart disease), and any drug sensitivities (especially to anesthetics). For instance, patients with a history of rheumatic heart disease, valvular heart disease, or cardiac lesions should receive prophylactic antibiotic therapy to protect them from the development of subacute bacterial endocarditis (SBE). A history of medications the woman is currently using should also be obtained to avoid therapeutic complications.

Treatment of incomplete abortion.   If the patient is presenting with an incomplete abortion initated elsewhere, she will often be bleeding heavily and require urgent examination and aspiration. The possibility of sepsis should always be considered and prophylactic antibiotics administered. The operator will usually find that the cervix is already well dilated in these patients.

Contraindications.   The patient's pregnancy history is of great importance in interpreting the findings of uterine size and in selection of the proper cannulas for sounding and aspiration. Acute pelvic pain, pelvic inflammatory disease (PID), a palpable pelvic mass or tenderness, anemia, disorders of blood coagulation, and known or suspected uterine fibroids may be contraindications to uterine aspiration on an outpatient basis (Table 5-3).

Ectopic pregnancy symptoms.   It is critical at this stage to attempt to screen out women presenting with symptoms of ectopic pregnancy. Ectopic or tubal pregnancies occur when the fertilized ovum implants before reaching the uterine cavity, usually in the fallopian tube. Ectopic pregnancies are rare (1 out of 200 total pregnancies, or 0.5%), but their consequences can be life-threatening. The group of symptoms that classically define ectopic pregnancy are: abnormal uterine bleeding, pelvic pain or tenderness, recent

Table 5-3. Contraindications to Outpatient Uterine Aspiration.
• Acute pelvic pain • Pelvic infection • Palpable pelvic mass or tenderness • Anemia • Uterine fibroids • Blood coagulation disorders

Table 5-4.
Symptoms of Ectopic Pregnancy.
• Abnormal uterine bleeding • Pelvic pain or tenderness (especially after first year of IUD use) • Palpable adnexal mass or tenderness • Recent spotting

spotting, and a palpable adnexal mass or tenderness (Table 5-4). (The adnexa include the ovaries, tubes, and uterine ligaments.) Few patients present with *all* these symptoms and unfortunately many ectopic pregnancies are entirely asymptomatic. It is important to listen carefully to the patient's description of her recent menstrual history and experience with this present pregnancy. When was her last *normal* menstrual period? Her most recent bleeding episode may have been spotting rather than menstruation, which, combined with other symptoms and an adnexal mass, would raise the suspicion of ectopic pregnancy.

If the examiner finds a palpable adnexal mass or tenderness, accompanied by a history of most of the symptoms listed above, the woman should be immediately referred to a health facility that is prepared to accurately diagnose and treat ectopic pregnancy. *Both* an adnexal mass *and* other symptoms are necessary for an absolute contraindication to uterine aspiration. If no adnexal mass accompanies the other symptoms, or if a mass is present without other symptoms, the possibility of ectopic pregnancy is remote and the aspiration can proceed.

Since it is common for patients with ectopic pregnancy to have exhibited no symptoms before aspirations, the aspirate must be inspected closely immediately after the procedure (see page 203).

Physical Examination

A general physical examination should be done on every woman seeking menstrual induction. Although it is not necessary that the examination be exhaustive, it should include auscultation of the heart and lungs and determination of blood pressure. Breasts, abdomen, and extremities should also be examined.

Bimanual pelvic examination. The pelvic examination should be conducted after the bladder has been emptied. Bimanual examination should determine the size, shape, and position of the uterus

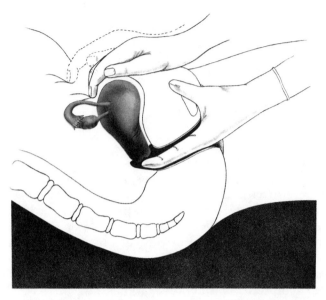

Figure 5-13. *Bimanual pelvic examination. By sweeping the abdominal hand towards the pubic bone, the examiner can palpate the uterine fundus and estimate its size.*

as well as cervical and uterine texture, judging their appropriateness for the period of amenorrhea (Figure 5-13). If uterine size is disproportionately large, if there is a finding such as a mass or tenderness suggestive of a pregnancy outside the uterus, if there is inflammatory disease, or if any of these findings are suspected, the operator must be willing to abandon the procedure at this point.

With the patient on an examining table in the lithotomy position, the operator begins the bimanual examination by separating the labia minora and depressing the perineum with two fingers of a gloved hand. The fingers are gently introduced into the vagina until the cervix is reached. The fingers of the opposite hand stabilize the pelvic contents by means of gentle pressure through the abdominal wall. If gentle motion of the cervix or corpus causes the woman to feel tenderness or pain, there may be acute or chronic inflammation. Such findings may also raise the suspicion of ectopic pregnancy when combined with other symptoms.

With the vaginal fingers stabilizing the cervix as a reference point, the uterine fundus is palpated by placing the other hand on the upper abdomen and sweeping it toward the pubic bone. A normally positioned uterus can be felt between the two hands. If the uterus is retroflexed or retroverted, it may not be palpable from the abdomen, but can be felt by gently stretching the posterior vaginal vault with the examining finger. With the uterus thus between the two hands, the operator can make a fairly accurate estimation of uterine size (see below).

The bimanual examination should also include the ovaries and adnexa (see Figure 3-14). By placing both fingers of the vaginal hand on one adnexal side, and pressing with the abdominal hand, the ovary on that side can usually be felt. The normal fallopian tube will not be distinguishable. Gentleness is essential because the ovaries are usually distinctly tender. *Unusual* tenderness in the ovaries or other areas of the adnexa may indicate inflammation. Palpation of an unexpected fullness or mass may indicate ectopic pregnancy, uterine fibroids, an ovarian cyst, or pelvic malignancy. All require further investigation before proceeding with uterine aspiration.

Uterine size, position, and consistency. A rough estimation of the duration of gestation can be made by assessing uterine size. When pregnancy occurs, the *overall* uterine size increases, but in the first weeks the increment is almost imperceptible. The first increases in size are limited to a slight change in the depth of the cavity, and then the corpus takes on a fully rounded shape. At 42 days LMP the size increase is usually so slight as to be easily overlooked. The globular shape of the uterus may be a distinctive diagnostic clue.

At about this time the softening of the lower uterine segment becomes palpable to an examiner. The cervix becomes softer and rather boggy, and the corpus takes on a somewhat doughy consistency. The area between the cervix and the corpus called the *isthmus* becomes so soft as to make the uterus seem discontinuous and excessively flexible. The relative firmness of the cervix, when followed upward with the internal examining hand, disappears into a soft connecting link with the fundus. This is called *Hegar's sign* and is most valuable in diagnosing early pregnancy (Figure 5-14).

As uterine size increases, the fundus rises from its normal nonpregnant position within the pelvis to an abdominal location. This usually occurs when the diameter of the fundus exceeds 8 cm, at about 70 days LMP. When the uterus has risen into the abdomen, it should be palpable as an abdominal organ just above the pubic bone.

Determining the position of the uterus at pelvic examination is essential to the interpretation of uterine size and to proper insertion of the aspiration cannula. A uterus that is sharply retroverted may be palpable, but the size of the retroverted uterus is often underesti-

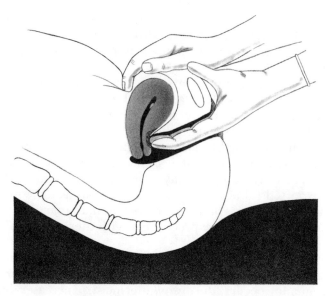

Figure 5-14. *Hegar's sign—when the uterine isthmus feels discontinuous—is an early sign of pregnancy.*

mated. A uterus that has a milder degree of retroversion may be impossible to outline on bimanual examination, and a rectovaginal examination should be employed to gain as much information about uterine size and texture as possible.

Estimating uterine size and correlating that estimate with the history of amenorrhea is not an easy task. Since the uterine fundus tends to take on a globular shape after 42 days LMP, the examiner should try to estimate the uterine diameter. Unfortunately, these measurements tend to be very subjective and vary from patient to patient and from examiner to examiner. This portion of the examination requires experience and persistence. Even skilled examiners sometimes have difficulty. Audiovisual training materials can help (see page xiii), but "hands-on" training under close supervision is mandatory.

Rather than limiting descriptions of the uterus to mathematical terms, examiners sometimes prefer to relate the uterine size to that of common fruits. Obviously, fruits also vary from place to place in both size and availability. Nevertheless, for some practitioners, it is useful to relate the nonpregnant uterus to the shape of a pear, the 42-day uterus to the size of a tangerine, and the 56-day uterus to the size of a small orange. Carrying this analogy further, the 70-day uterus can be compared to a large orange, the 12-week uterus to a grapefruit, and the 14-week uterus to a small melon.

If the pregnancy is estimated to be advanced beyond 50 days LMP, in order to proceed the examiner must be trained and equipped to provide suction curettage or otherwise refer the patient to an appropriate facility.

Examination of the vagina and cervix.   After the examiner completes bimanual uterine palpation and is satisfied that the patient qualifies for an aspiration procedure that the operator is able to provide, the physical examination is continued. The external genitalia and the introitus are inspected and a speculum inserted into the vagina. The character of the vaginal and cervical secretions are then noted. If vaginal infection appears possible, a wet preparation of the vaginal secretions should be examined so that proper treatment can proceed after the aspiration. If cervicitis is evident or if gonorrhea is suspected, a cervical culture or a Gram stain smear of cervical secretions should be obtained. Unless cervical and vaginal infections are severe or specific therapy is not available, they need not be considered contraindications to uterine aspiration.

The external cervical os will appear distinctly different to the examiner depending on the woman's parity and general health. If the woman has never delivered a baby vaginally, the os is likely to have a round or very slightly flattened shape. If parous, the os is likely to be more like a transverse slit with slight mobility of the top and bottom lips. If the cervix has been previously lacerated, it may be more distorted, with multiple slits radiating from the central portion of the os. In early pregnancy the cervix has a slightly blue color and a soft texture. This has often been compared to the texture of the skin over the chin; in the nonpregnant state the cervix has been compared to the texture of the tip of the nose.

The mucus within the cervical canal can reveal important diagnostic clues and should be carefully observed. The consistency of this mucus is dependent on the hormonal state of the woman. In the highly estrogenic preovulatory state, most women have an increased amount of cervical mucus, sometimes of sufficient quantity that it produces a symptomatic vaginal discharge. Such estrogenic mucus takes on a stringy character in the absence of progesterone. If grasped with an instrument, it may pull out in sticky threads of up to 10 cm in length. This characteristic is called *spinnbarkeit* and is not seen in early pregnancy because it is eliminated by circulating progesterone.

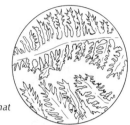

Figure 5-15. *A microscopic examination of cervical mucus that shows ferning crystals is inconsistent with pregnancy.*

When cervical mucus that is highly estrogenic and without progesterone is spread on a microscope slide and allowed to dry in the air, it takes on a peculiar crystalline form called *ferning*—crystals in the shape of fern leaves (Figure 5-15). As progesterone levels rise after ovulation, ferning disappears. The finding of spinnbarkeit and ferning is inconsistent with pregnancy; the absence of these findings however, does *not* necessarily *prove* pregnancy.

Preparation of the Patient

The procedure begins with the patient lying down on the treatment table and assuming the lithotomy position: lying on her back with her legs open, raised, bent at the knee and resting on the supports.

Prior to any instrumentation or injection in the cervical or vaginal tissues, the area is cleansed with an antiseptic solution. The antiseptic is applied with a cotton ball held by forceps. The surface of the cervix should be cleaned and the excess mucus in the external os wiped away. The vaginal vault should also be cleaned, especially if an anesthetic injection will be used. Benzalkonium chloride 1:750 or a providone–iodine solution is suitable for this purpose, as are other products that may be available to the practitioner.

At this point in the procedural preparation, the operator is at a critical stage and must stop and evaluate the patient's suitability for uterine aspiration and the technique chosen—menstrual induction or suction curettage. After proper adequate counseling either by the operator or a designated counselor, having performed those laboratory determinations appropriate to the patient and the clinic, having completed a basic physical examination and history, having administered antibiotics to patients with suspected septic incomplete abortion, and having not found any contraindications, the operator is now ready to proceed with the first *active* step in the procedure.

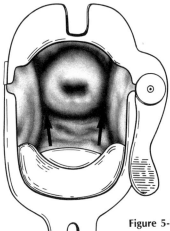

Figure 5-16. *A paracervical block is advised for most menstrual induction procedures.*

Anesthesia. The need for anesthesia varies with the pain threshold of the patient and skill of the operator. Menstrual induction can often be done without anesthesia, but if the patient indicates discomfort or fear of pain either before or after the cannula insertion begins, a paracervical block is well advised. General anesthesia is *not* appropriate except in rare circumstances; its use unnecessarily causes a two- to fourfold increase in the risk of death from first-trimester abortion.

If a paracervical block is used, the cervix is first stabilized with the tenaculum. The anesthetic is injected at 4 o'clock and 8 o'clock positions into the upper vaginal wall alongside the cervix at an approximate depth of 0.5 cm beneath the vaginal surface (Figure 5-16).

Lidocaine hydrochloride 1%, 5 ml on each side, is frequently used, although there are many other suitable medications. Before injection the provider must make sure that the patient is not allergic to the medication chosen. Care must be taken to avoid injection into a blood vessel. After the injection, it is wise to wait briefly while anesthesia becomes established. During that interval the syringe and cannula can be prepared for the aspiration procedure.

Menstrual Induction: Pregnancies Less than 50 Days LMP

Assembly. The syringe should now be assembled and "charged" (Figure 5-17). It is advisable to "charge" a second syringe at the same time so as to have it quickly available if vacuum should

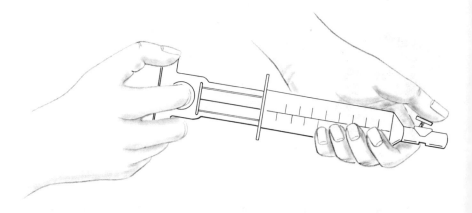

Figure 5-17. *The menstrual induction syringe is charged by pushing forward on the pinch valve to close it and then withdrawing the plunger to create the vacuum.*

be lost in the first syringe, or if the volume of aspirate exceeds expectations.

To charge the syringe:

1. Close the pinch valve by pushing the cap down and forward with the thumb.
2. Withdraw the plunger the full length of the syringe until the locking handles are engaged against the base of the syringe.

When ready for aspiration, the syringe's connecting adaptor is attached to the end of the cannula (already inserted in the uterus—see below).

A decision must be made regarding the size of the cannula that is to be used for aspiration. Under usual circumstances the sizes shown in Table 5-5 are appropriate, but the selection depends on the practitioner's experience, preference, and techniques of aspiration. Most often, the 4-mm cannula is used only as a uterine sound and aspiration is performed with the 5- or 6-mm cannula.

It is not necessary to use sterile gloves for this procedure, but use of a sterile "no touch" technique is mandatory. In this technique, that portion of the sterile cannula that will enter the uterus is not touched by the hand, or by any unsterile object. If manipulation of that portion of the cannula becomes necessary the maneuver is

Table 5-5. Cannula Size and Gestational Age.	
Days LMP	Cannula Size (mm)
29–35	4
36–42	5
43–50	6

either done with a sterile instrument or the cannula is discarded and replaced by a fresh, sterile one.

Sounding. At 6 weeks LMP a parous cervix with a loose external os might well receive the 6-mm cannula directly with minimal resistance at the internal os. However, a nulliparous cervix may resist even the 4-mm cannula with initial instrumentation. In such cases the 4-mm cannula can usually be inserted by using persistent gentle pressure with a very slight torsion or twisting effort as the tip bears against the internal os. If by chance the cannula should buckle or kink with this effort, it can be grasped in its middle or distal portion with the polyp forceps and the effort reapplied with this instrument. Sounding is usually performed with the first cannula passed.

When the internal os has been negotiated, the uterine depth is sounded by inserting the cannula upward until the fundus is touched. The flexible cannula allows the fundus to be sensed with lessened danger of perforation since excessive pressure tends to fold or kink the instrument rather than to perforate the uterus.

The fundus is usually reached at a depth in centimeters roughly proportional to the length of amenorrhea in weeks (see Table 5-2), but considerable variation may be found in correlation with parity, uterine size, and the presence of pathological conditions of the uterus. Sounding to an excess depth would indicate three possibilities:

1. Error in gestational date, either by history or by misunderstanding of the bimanual examination
2. Unrecognized uterine disease (fibroids)
3. Uterine perforation (with flexible cannulas, this is a rare but possible hazard)

Any one of these three situations requires reconsideration of the aspiration procedure and referral for appropriate treatment.

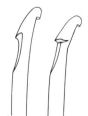

Figure 5-18. *Each aspiration cannula should be inspected prior to use to ensure that the notches are fully open and not cracked.*

Aspiration. Assuming that the sounding with the first cannula is appropriate, the next larger size can be inserted and if necessary, the next size in turn. For patients who are nulliparous or who have been amenorrheic for less than 40 days, a 5-mm cannula is usually satisfactory for aspiration. Otherwise, the 6-mm cannula is usually used. Whatever the size selected, the cannula that will be used for the actual aspiration should be carefully inspected by the operator. *Every* aspiration cannula should be inspected; even new cannulas are occasionally defective (Figure 5-18). The notches should be fully open, and the bridges between the upper and lower notches of the cannula side wall must be intact, with no signs of cracking or collapse.

As the aspiration cannula is inserted to the fundus, the operator must be careful to touch only the open end that connects to the syringe. This cannula should pass to the same depth as did the sounding cannula. Insertion of a cannula is usually done without the syringe attached in order to have maximum control in the maneuver. When the fundus is reached, the syringe is then attached and the vacuum released into the cannula by opening the pinch valve (Figure 5-19).

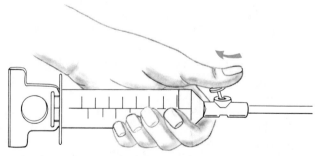

Figure 5-19. *After the syringe is attached, the vacuum is released into the cannula by pulling back and up on the pinch valve.*

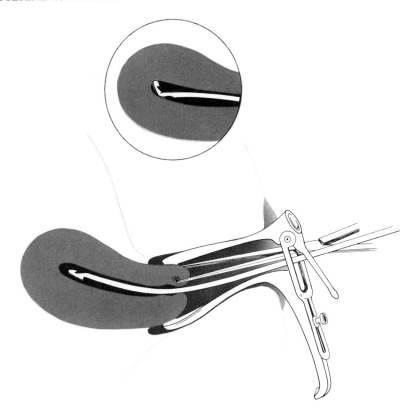

Figure 5-20. *Uterine aspiration is accomplished by very short in and out stroking motions of the cannula. Inset shows how the atraumatic plastic cannula will bend when it presses against the fundus, avoiding perforation.*

Accompanied by very short in and out stroking motions within the uterus (Figure 5-20) the cannula is rotated in the upper segment of the uterine cavity through a complete arc. This is best accomplished by (1) slowly rotating 180° in one direction; (2) reversing direction, returning to the starting position and rotating beyond it 180°; and then (3) reversing again and returning 180° to the starting position (Figure 5-21).

Some operators prefer to simply rotate in one direction with very short stroking action, progressing through at least two complete revolutions. This is a very effective method of emptying the uterine cavity but may cause fracture of the cannula tip and on rare occasions loss of the tip in the uterus. If the tip is ever lost in the

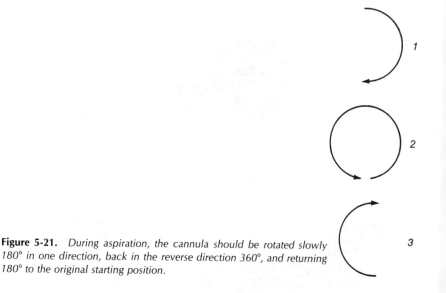

Figure 5-21. *During aspiration, the cannula should be rotated slowly 180° in one direction, back in the reverse direction 360°, and returning 180° to the original starting position.*

cavity, additional uterine instrumentation will be required for retrieval of the fragment.

The operator should be aware that the vacuum capacity of the syringe falls markedly when it is half filled with aspirate. When this occurs, the pinch valve should be closed and the syringe detached from the cannula. To empty the syringe, the pinch valve is reopened and the plunger depressed. The procedure can be continued after recharging the syringe and reconnecting it to the cannula.

When tissue flow in the cannula from the upper segment of the uterine cavity ceases or slows markedly, the in-and-out stroking motions are amplified to include the entire uterine wall, and the rotary motion is repeated. Special attention must be given at this time to the 2, 4, 8, and 10 o'clock positions, so that the cornual region of the cavity are completely aspirated.

The use of oxytocic agents in this procedure to induce contractions of the uterine muscle is necessary only in cases of uterine atony (failure of the uterus to contract) or grand multiparity. Oxytocics can precipitate as many problems as they solve. If they are needed, however, 0.25 mg of ergometrine or 0.2 mg of methylergonovine may be used intramuscularly during or immediately after the procedure.

If a simple lack of tissue flow in the cannula is observed *without* the appearance of tiny air bubbles, one assumes that blockage of the cannula by tissue fragments has occurred. The cannula should be removed and inspected. If a tissue fragment is adhering to one of the notches, it can be brushed away with a sterile sponge. The cannula can then be reinserted if no contamination has occurred, but it is probably better to simply begin the aspiration procedure anew with a fresh, sterile cannula and a freshly charged syringe. Whenever the procedure is interrupted, the rule that *the plunger of the syringe is manipulated ONLY when the cannula is disconnected* must always be followed. One must never allow aspirate to be forced back into either the cannula or the uterus, nor should air ever be forced back into the uterine cavity.

The procedure is considered complete when:

1. Small bubbles (red foam) are seen in the cannula and no further tissue flow can be elicited by motion of the instrument.
2. The characteristic gritty vibration of the cannula against the evacuated uterine wall is sensed.
3. A strong uterine contraction can be felt gripping the cannula, making continued aspiration difficult.

If the slightest doubt exists about the completeness of the aspiration of the uterine contents, it is wise to reaspirate, using a cannula one size *smaller* than that used for the first aspiration. When the operator is satisfied that the criteria of completion have been fulfilled, the cannula is removed. If the woman has chosen to use an IUD, it is inserted at this time.

Inspection of aspirate.   The aspirate can be easily inspected by ejecting the aspirate from the syringe into a wire strainer and rinsing out the bloody fluid. The solid tissue remaining can then be inspected closely, or floated in a small glass vessel filled with saline solution. The fingerlike projections of the chorionic villi can be recognized in this manner. A hand lens or reading glass may assist in visualization of the villi. The absence of villi may indicate incomplete aspiration, ectopic pregnancy, or other causes of amenorrhea (see page 209).

The operator should also check the total volume of the aspirate obtained. Too little tissue for the estimated gestational age is another warning sign for ectopic pregnancy (see page 190). Excessive tissue may indicate hydatidiform mole, and a pathological examination of the aspirate would then be mandatory.

The entire procedure usually takes 5–15 minutes. The patient is ordinarily allowed to rest on the treatment table for a few minutes after the aspiration during examination of the aspirate. Ordinarily she should be observed for 30 minutes and allowed to leave when her vital signs are stable and she has been given her follow-up instructions.

Suction Curettage:
Pregnancies Beyond 50 Days LMP

In the event that a woman seeking uterine aspiration presents a history that is found to exceed 50 days LMP, or if on examination she is found to exceed the limits of uterine size for menstrual induction, or if her uterus sounds to a depth that would indicate that the gestational age exceeds 50 days, the practitioner must make the difficult and critical decision of whether or not to proceed. The procedure preparation should be stopped if the practitioner is not a physician with both the skills and the facilities necessary to proceed with an evacuation requiring significant cervical dilation. Immediate referral to an appropriately skilled physician is necessary.

On the other hand, provided the practitioner has the skills and the proper equipment, aspiration techniques can be used in an outpatient setting to evacuate a uterus considerably more advanced in gestational age than 50 days. Indeed, despite the most rigorous efforts to conservatively screen patients by taking the history, examination, and sounding, aspiration nevertheless may be mistakenly attempted in a patient who should have been rejected for menstrual induction. Consequently, unless an appropriate referral facility is easily available, the provider should be capable of coping with a more advanced pregnancy.

In these situations a cannula larger than 6 mm in diameter will be required. After 50 days LMP, the cannula diameter required is approximately equal to 1 mm per week of gestation (Table 5-6). That is, an 8-mm cannula is used at 56 days LMP (8 weeks), a 10-mm cannula at 70 days (10 weeks), and a 12-mm cannula at 12 weeks.

If cannulas larger than 6 mm are used, two adaptations of the vacuum source are required. The total volume of the vacuum must be adequate for the uterine contents to be aspirated, and the pinch-valve connector must be able to accept the larger diameter of the aspirating cannula. It is important to realize that the 6-mm cannula is the largest size appropriate for the connector supplied with the menstrual induction syringe. Larger syringes or electric vacuum aspirators can accommodate larger-size cannulas for more advanced pregnancies.

Table 5-6. Cervical Dilation and Gestational Age.				
Week LMP	Sounding Depth (cm)	Cannula Size (mm)	Pratt Dilator (no.)	Hegar Dilator (no.)
7½–8	8–9	8	25	9
9–10	10–11	10	31–33	11–12
11–12	12–13	12	37–39	13–14

The preparation of the patient and the administration of paracervical anesthesia are performed in the same way for suction curettage patients as for menstrual induction patients. Since suction curettage is probably more often used than menstrual induction in the treatment of incomplete abortion, the operator must remember to consider the possibility of sepsis and administer prophylactic antibiotics if indicated.

After waiting a few minutes for the anesthesia to take effect, the uterus is carefully sounded to determine the depth and direction of the cervical canal. The depth of sounding for any given gestational age can vary, but generally it will be 1–2 cm greater than the gestational age in weeks LMP: a uterus of 10 weeks' gestational age will sound to 11 or perhaps 12 cm. A uterus sounding to more than 13 cm is likely to be more than 12 weeks' gestational age.

Dilation.   Dilation must be accomplished to an opening slightly larger than the cannula to be used. This is necessary to allow the cannula free motion within the cervical canal. The cervical tissues are very elastic at this gestational age and begin to close back rather quickly, making free cannula motion difficult if some overdilation is not achieved.

Pratt dilators are preferable instruments for dilation, because of their ideal curve, gradual taper, and small increments in size from one to another. The numbers on the dilators are roughly *three times* their diameter in millimeters. Hegar dilators can also be used; they are calibrated in millimeters of *actual* diameter (Table 5-6). Pratt and Hegar dilators are metallic; new Teflon dilators (Denniston dilators) are also well suited for use in suction currettage and are less expensive than the metal instruments.

With the cervix stabilized by a tenaculum, the smallest-size dilator is gently inserted in the axis of the cervical canal to a point beyond the internal os. Usually, the no. 17 Pratt can be inserted without resistance, but if resistance is encountered, one should begin the procedure with the no. 15 or no. 13. Gentleness and caution are essential. The next-larger-size dilator is passed, and then each succeeding size, one after the other, until the desired dilation is reached. Each dilator is passed to the same depth of sounding. When resistance is met, gentle and persistent pressure should be exerted, being *certain* that the force is applied only in the axis (previously sounded) of the cervical canal, and to a depth of only 1 or 2 cm beyond the internal os. The process should not be hurried. The dilator, once passed, should be allowed to remain in place for several seconds before being removed and replaced by the next in the series.

When the necessary opening has been achieved, the cannula is inserted. Cannulas used in suction curettage have their depth of sounding clearly marked in the plastic. This indicator should be watched carefully. The entire cannula opening must be within the uterine cavity, but the tip need *not* reach the fundus. Knowing the depth of the internal os and the depth of sounding makes it easier for the operator to judge this placement.

Aspiration.   The vacuum source is then attached to the cannula, and the pinch valve is opened. (On those systems that operate with a control handle rather than a pinch valve, the vacuum relief vent is *closed* at this point to apply the vacuum to the cannula.)

The vacuum being applied to the cannula should be greater than 60 mm (25 in.) Hg. An immediate flow of fluid and placental tissues should be noted. The cannula is then gently and systematically rotated completely around the uterine cavity, and then short in-and-out motions are added. In this fashion, the entire endometrial surface can be cleaned of placental and decidual tissues.

Occasionally, and especially if gestational age is greater than estimated, tissue fragments may be too large to pass through the cannula. In such a case, slow and careful work with the cannula— removing it, clearing it of obstruction, and reinserting it and reaspirating (repeatedly if necessary)—will bring the larger fragments into the lower uterine segment, where they can be removed by the forceps.

As the uterus empties, it begins to contract forcibly, and the cavity becomes less deep. Sensing this contraction is important to avoid perforation with the cannula. This contraction is also a desirable hemostatic mechanism. It is occasionally advantageous to

stimulate contraction with intravenous oxytocin, or another oxytocic drug.

When the operator feels secure that all tissue has been removed,
the cannula is removed and the cervix observed for a moment for
evidence of more than the usual uterine bleeding. If excessive bleeding occurs, one should be suspicious of retained tissues. Reaspiration or exploration of the cavity with a sharp metal curette may be
necessary. Incomplete removal of the products of conception is a
major cause of postoperative hemorrhage and infection, and the
operator must take every reasonable precaution to see that no tissue
remains.

The total volume of aspirate in relation to estimated gestational age must be noted, as in menstrual induction. Too little
tissue may indicate ectopic pregnancy (see page 190); too much
may indicate hydatidiform mole, requiring pathological examination of the aspirate.

FOLLOW-UP

Patient Instructions

Immediate postprocedure instructions to the patient are directed toward providing her a comfortable, speedy recovery without
excessive bleeding or development of infection:

1. The patient should refrain from heavy work or vigorous physical
   activity for a day or two; however, she need not be confined to
   bed or be treated as an invalid.
2. She may require mild analgesics if she is particularly sensitive to
   uterine cramps.
3. She should refrain from sexual intercourse and from douching
   for several days.
4. She should report for follow-up examination in 1–2 weeks.

In order that she not experience excessive anxiety because of the
occurrence of expected postprocedure symptoms, the patient should
be informed of the following facts:

1. The presence of fever is abnormal. If she develops a temperature
   of 38°C (100.4°F) or more or has chills, lassitude, or other symp-

toms of febrile illness, she should contact her practitioner for appropriate therapy. Women treated for incomplete abortion should be monitored even more carefully for signs of postoperative infection.

2. Some bleeding is to be expected. It should be as much *but not more than* that experienced in a normal menstrual period. A light intermittent flow may persist as much as 10 days after the procedure. Excessive bleeding or the passage of significant clots warrant return to the clinic and possible reaspiration.

3. Mild cramping pain is expected. Severe pain is not, and should be reported. Cramping may be a bit more pronounced if an IUD has been inserted.

4. Symptoms of pregnancy such as breast soreness or nausea may continue up to 7 days after uterine aspiration. If they persist beyond that time, the patient should report back for an examination and possible reaspiration. If the woman began taking oral contraceptives immediately after the procedure, however, remember that their side-effects may mimic pregnancy in some women.

5. A normal menstrual period should begin within 4–6 weeks. Again, the method of contraception accepted by the patient and its regimen must be taken into account.

Postprocedure contraception.   Encouragement for postaspiration contraceptive use is an essential part of the complete procedure. The woman must realize that her fertility can return almost immediately after aspiration. All contraceptive methods are suitable for women who have just completed menstrual induction. Oral contraceptives or injectable contraceptives may be started immediately after the procedure. Intrauterine devices may be inserted immediately after the procedure while the patient is still in the treatment room or at the time of the first follow-up visit. If a woman selects the diaphragm as her contraceptive method, it can be fitted immediately after the procedure, but it is more advisable to wait until the first follow-up visit for diaphragm fitting. Uterine aspiration does not in any way affect a woman's medical eligibility for a sterilization procedure, and it can be performed concurrently if desired. Because of the psychological stress surrounding a pregnancy termination procedure, however, this is not always the best time for the patient to make a sterilization decision.

Complications and Management

Fewer than 1% of all uterine aspiration patients experience serious complications. According to the U.S. Centers for Disease Control (CDC), the risk of mortality due to uterine aspiration is actually lower than the risk following tonsillectomy. Nevertheless, the practitioner must be able to recognize the possible complications of uterine aspiration. Some of these complications are minor problems that can be resolved in the same clinical setting and by the same personnel as the original procedure. Other conditions may require referral to a more sophisticated setting or to physicians with more training.

The two major possible complications are *incomplete aspiration*, when the pregnancy is terminated, but some products of conception remain, and *failed termination*, when the pregnancy continues. Other uterine aspiration complications include failure of the uterus to contract after the procedure, cervical or uterine trauma, and the effects caused by products of conception that were degenerating before the procedure began. Researchers in numerous clinical studies have determined that the overall incidence of these complications after uterine aspiration is around 5% or less of all cases (see page 216).

Incomplete aspiration. Interruption of pregnancy with incomplete removal of the products of conception can result in excessive bleeding or intrauterine infection, and usually both. The common causes of such incomplete aspiration are either that the procedure was incompletely evacuated and not all the endometrial surface was cleaned by the cannula, or that a cannula was used that was too small for the gestational age. The problem can usually be handled by reaspiration with a cannula appropriate to the size of the uterus. If this fails, the patient should have a conventional dilation and curettage. Febrile patients with incomplete aspirations or previously induced incomplete abortions should be considered as septic and treated with appropriate antibiotics as well.

There is an extremely rare but theoretically possible outcome of incomplete aspiration—the remaining placental tissues could undergo abnormal growth. This is what is called *trophoblastic disease*. These growths can be benign or malignant and include hydatidiform mole, chorioadenoma, and choriocarcinoma. If curettage is used to treat a postabortal patient for persistent bleeding or spotting, the tissue must be submitted for examination by a pathologist to rule out trophoblastic disease.

Failed termination. If the cannula selected for aspiration was too small, or the uterus aspirated was too large, an intrauterine implantation site may remain intact and continue to develop. Unfortunately, failure occurs more often (in up to 5% of all procedures) when uterine aspiration is attempted too early in pregnancy. Therefore, the aspiration procedure should usually be delayed until after 35 days LMP, when the period is a week or more late. Even when aspirating women between 35 and 42 days LMP, operators should be certain that the uterus is empty by sensing the "uterine cry"—the curettelike scraping of the cannula on the uterine wall—in all segments of the cavity.

Failure to terminate can be suspected immediately by the inspection of the aspirated material (see page 203). If no chorionic villi are discovered, three distinct possibilities must come to mind:

1. The patient may not have been pregnant.
2. The patient may have an ectopic pregnancy.
3. The patient may have a deformed uterus.

In situation 1 a small amount of endometrial tissue has probably been obtained. When examined microscopically, no decidua would be seen in this sample. Menstrual induction procedures have frequently been criticized because of the relative frequency of aspirating patients who are not pregnant although their period is 1 or 2 weeks late. Clinical studies (see page 217) have found this occurring in 30%–40% of women before 35 days LMP and less than 20% between 35 and 42 days LMP. The undesirability of cannula aspiration in a nonpregnant patient, however, is sometimes outweighed by the reassurance the aspiration provides to a woman who does not wish to be pregnant.

An ectopic pregnancy (situation 2, above) occurs when the fertilized egg is developing outside the uterine cavity—usually in the fallopian tube. Ectopic pregnancies are rare: in a study of 55,000 abortions performed in Washington, D.C., over a 5-year period, only 22 cases were seen. But they are dangerous: the mortality rate from ectopic pregnancy in the United States overall was estimated at 1 death per 1000 cases in 1978; it is assumed to be much higher in developing countries. This mortality rate is five times as high in abortion-revealed cases because a normal pregnancy is usually first assumed, delaying the diagnosis of ectopic pregnancy.

When no chorionic villi are found in the aspirate (especially after 42 days LMP), when the pregnancy test was positive or not clearly negative, and when a history of other symptoms was presented (adnexal mass or irregular bleeding; see page 190), the patient should be immediately referred to an appropriate facility. The management of ectopic pregnancy requires a well-equipped operating room and skilled physicians.

The aspirated tissue must also be sent to the referral source for urgent pathological examination. If proliferative or secretory endometrium are found, the patient is not pregnant and will be released. If no endometrial tissue is found at all, a repeat pregnancy test and close monitoring will be sufficient. If decidua or hypersecretory endometrium (Arias-Stella phenomena) are found, ectopic pregnancy will be assumed and laparoscopy initiated.

A failed termination could occur because of an abnormality in uterine structure (situation 3, above). Congenital malformations of the uterus are not infrequent and range from an exaggerated wideness of the uterine cavity (*arcuate* uterus) to the presence of two

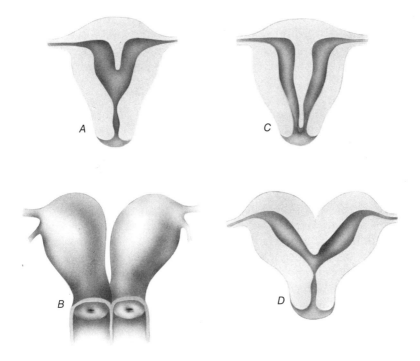

Figure 5-22. *Undetected congenital malformations of the uterus can cause a failed termination of pregnancy. Shown are arcuate (A), didelphic (B), septate (C), and bicornuate (D) uteri.*

complete uteri (*didelphic* uterus). In these two extremes few problems should be encountered by the careful operator. The arcuate uterus (Figure 5-22A) will usually be completely emptied when the standard aspiration technique is used. The presence of a didelphic uterus (Figure 5-22B) should be evident because the careful operator will see two cervices, or sometimes even a double vagina.

The *septate* uterus (Figure 5-22C), which is outwardly normal but has an internal septum or divider, and the *bicornuate* uterus (Figure 5-22D), which has a cavity with two separate horns connected to a single cervix, present the problem of two cavities to aspirate. In all likelihood only one of these cavities will be entered by the aspirating cannula, and the contents of the other cavity will be left undisturbed.

If the undisturbed cavity contains only decidua, some protracted bleeding will occur, but usually will relent spontaneously. If the undisturbed portion of the uterus contains the implantation site, however, the termination procedure will have failed and the pregnancy will continue. Should the uterus feel irregular or asymmetrically enlarged on bimanual examination, or if only decidua is obtained by aspiration and ectopic pregnancy has been ruled out, a malformation of the uterus should be expected and the patient reexamined.

Other bleeding complications. Although retained tissue is by far the most common reason for postabortal bleeding, it is not the only cause. In some unusual cases the uterine muscle has difficulty in initiating or maintaining firm contraction (*uterine atony*), resulting in a failure of the endometrial blood vessels in the denuded implantation site to close off. Bleeding will continue until firm contraction of the uterus is achieved. This can usually be managed by the administration of an oxytocic agent such as an ergot derivative or by manual massage of the uterus.

One must also be aware that bleeding may occur as a result of unrecognized cervical or uterine trauma. *Cervical tears* can result from too much tension on the tenaculum, or even the tenaculum's grip itself may on occasion cause some troublesome bleeding. These cervical injuries should be looked for immediately after the procedure, and can be repaired by suture if necessary.

Uterine perforation, though very rare in menstrual induction, is nevertheless possible. Perforation can occur more often in suction curettage cases, and may happen during sounding, dilation or cannula manipulation. Perforation may be more likely in women with

Table 5-7. Symptoms of Uterine Perforation.
• Abnormal bleeding
• Falling hematocrit
• Abdominal pain
• Abdominal distention or ileus
• Fever
• Destabilization of pulse and blood pressure

an unusually rigid cervical canal, or in those whose uterus is sharply displaced or distorted from previous surgery, injury or disease. Perforations can be dangerous and proper care must be initiated at once.

The symptoms of perforation are variable and dependent on the site. Six symptoms are commonly encountered; all or none may be present (see also Table 5-7):

1. Abnormal bleeding from the cervix or vagina.
2. A falling hematocrit may indicate undetected abdominal bleeding.
3. Abdominal pain.
4. Abdominal distention or *ileus* (paralysis of the bowel) may indicate bowel injury from the perforation.
5. Fever.
6. Destabilization of pulse and blood pressure.

Although bleeding is the most common symptom, it is not unusual for none of these symptoms to appear at first. At other times, vaginal or abdominal bleeding may be profuse; these patients are at grave risk and require immediate referral for surgical intervention.

All patients in whom perforation is known or suspected require careful observation for 12–24 hours and referral for hospital care when necessary. If uterine perforation occurs when a large-diameter suction cannula is used, exploratory laparotomy (abdominal surgery) is mandatory *if* injury to the bowel or mesentery (connecting membrane) is suspected.

Missed abortion is a rare cause of bleeding associated with uterine aspiration. A missed abortion occurs when a pregnancy has begun to degenerate spontaneously before instrumentation of the uterus. If the uterus is incompletely aspirated, the remaining products of conception are necrotic (dying) and are a fertile medium for the growth of pathogenic bacteria. In some circumstances retained necrotic tissue may cause a clotting defect (afibrinogenemia) that results in widespread bleeding. This condition requires the services of a highly trained medical specialist. The disorder can be suspected when bleeding fails to form clots, bleeding develops from other body orifices or into the skin, and the products of conception are recognized as being necrotic or degenerated.

Effect on subsequent pregnancies. Several large-scale studies in the United States and elsewhere have been conducted to determine whether first-trimester elective abortion has an adverse effect on a woman's subsequent pregnancies. Eight separate studies, including one involving 32,000 women in California, have found that a history of prior induced abortion was *not* related to low birthweight, prematurity, spontaneous abortion (stillbirth), or other adverse outcomes when modern techniques involving *minimal cervical dilation* were used.

Two studies—one from Hungary and one from the United States—did find very small increased risks but found the effects of tobacco smoking on pregnancy outcomes to be many times worse. A 1979 Boston study found an association between a history of *repeated* first-trimester abortion and poor outcome in subsequent pregnancies but did *not* find a relationship to *single* previous abortions.

A 1982 Boston study found that women who have had two or more induced abortions have a relative risk of 2.6 that a subsequent pregnancy will be ectopic. A study of 17,000 women in Hawaii found no significant increase in poor outcome *regardless* of the number of previous induced abortions. Instead, a key risk factor was found to be the *interval* between the induced abortion and the subsequent pregnancy: if the interval is less than 1 year, the woman is much more likely to experience a spontaneous abortion.

The U.S. Centers for Disease Control (CDC), on reviewing these experiences, concluded that variations from study to study were probably due to difference in procedural technique and operator skill. Nevertheless, the CDC recommends that to help minimize any effect on subsequent pregnancies, providers should:

- Avoid sharp curettage.
- Avoid mechanical dilation over 11 mm.
- Advise patients to stop smoking.
- Counsel patients to leave a "sufficient" length of time—apparently 1 year or more—after an induced abortion before attempting a wanted pregnancy.

In summary, a single induced abortion, when performed by using one of the techniques described in this chapter, does not significantly affect a subsequent pregnancy. Repeat abortions—regardless of whether they contribute to poor subsequent pregnancy outcome—are clearly undesirable. Providers must therefore encourage their patients to not only accept an effective method of contraception after their uterine aspiration procedure, but also to *continue* to use it.

The CDC suggests that an even more conservative approach can be taken. If repeat abortions can affect the outcome of a subsequent wanted pregnancy, the nulliparous woman who eventually wants to have children should set her priority on *effectiveness* when choosing a contraceptive method. This approach would point toward the use of oral contraceptives (if not contraindicated), a combination of condoms and spermicidal foam, or perhaps very careful use of the diaphragm, in order to avoid repeated terminations of unwanted pregnancies.

CURRENT EXPERIENCE

It is now estimated that legally or illegally, 55 million women around the world seek abortions every year—about 150,000 per day. Reduction of the risks involved in this procedure can have a tremendous effect on the health and well-being of a significant number of the world's women. Condemning abortion as undesirable, and ignoring its unfortunate but necessary frequency, will not make abortion go away. It is a common experience for many women all over the world, and refinement of abortion techniques is of critical importance to public health.

Data compiled by the CDC show that the mortality rate for uterine aspiration procedures performed by modern techniques is less than for tonsillectomies. The rate is, in fact, much lower than the risk of dying associated with pregnancy. For pregnant adolescents, the contrast is particularly stark: childbearing holds a five times greater risk of death than a first-trimester abortion (9.5 deaths per 100,000 live births versus 1.8 deaths per 100,000 abortions).

Suction Curettage

Approximately 1.5 million abortions were performed in the United States alone in 1979, and most of them were performed by uterine aspiration in the first trimester. Literally hundreds of thou-

Study	Number of cases	Complication Rate(%)*	Failure Rate(%)†
Bozorgi 1977	12,219	0.7	0.02
Wulff 1977	16,410	1.5	0.5
Grimes 1979	66,763	0.7	n.a.

Table 5-8.
Selected Suction Curettage Clinical Studies.

*Complication rates include bleeding, pain, fever, infection, and retained products of conception.
†Failure rates are the rate of continuing pregnancy.

sands of suction curettage cases (sometimes referred to in the literature as *vacuum aspiration*) have been documented. The efficacy and safety of these procedures is impressive. For example, Table 5-8 lists three recent reports of clinical experience in the United States with suction curettage, totaling over 95,000 cases.

Menstrual Induction

Several million menstrual induction procedures have been performed worldwide. One estimate is that 5 million procedures were performed between 1974 and 1978. Over 20,000 cases have been documented in the literature (Table 5-9).

Complications (in abortion research, usually defined as any undesirable conditions caused by the procedure) are universally found to be less than 5%. Serious complications occur in less than 1% of procedures. Most complications are easily managed by well-prepared clinics and operators. Uterine perforations or cervical lacerations have a very low incidence.

Published studies report that the complete procedure usually lasts less than 10 minutes and blood loss is usually much less than

Table 5-9.
Menstrual Induction Clinical Studies.

Total number of cases documented	22,431
Number of studies	12
Study population sizes (range)	137–12,888
Complication rates (range)	0.8%–4.7%
Failure rates (range)	0–4.4%

50 ml. Most of the problems experienced by women having menstrual induction stem from a preexisting condition in the patient—pelvic inflammatory disease (PID), uterine fibroids, or incomplete abortion.

Effectiveness.   The effectiveness of the procedure—the success in removing the products of conception completely—has usually been found to be at least 95%, with reaspiration the usual solution to incomplete abortion. It is also clear from clinical studies that procedural success increases sharply after 35 days LMP.

Nonphysician providers.   In many places, nonphysician health providers have been trained to perform menstrual inductions under medical supervision. One 1977–1978 study conducted in Bangladesh, where paramedical providers perform menstrual inductions up to 9 weeks LMP, yielded an overall complication rate of 1.4%, comparable to previously reported rates achieved by physicians. Another 1976 study of nonphysician providers showed a similar complication rate of 1.3%. Nonphysician delivery of menstrual induction can be a critically important means of spreading the availability of this health service. With training, experience, and adequate backup facilities, menstrual induction is an extremely safe means of pregnancy termination.

Postprocedure contraception.   Studies of menstrual induction have also clearly demonstrated that a woman seeking interruption of pregnancy is highly motivated to accept contraception. In 1975, the International Fertility Research Program (IFRP) reported that, according to data it was receiving from providers worldwide, the number of women using a highly effective contraceptive method (pills, IUDs, injectables, or sterilization) before menstrual induction averaged 13%. After the procedure the figure rose to 51%. A 1977–1978 review of data reported to The Pathfinder Fund showed a similar pattern. Among women receiving menstrual inductions in five separate studies, 40% were using a contraceptive method prior to the procedure, whereas 92% were using a method afterward; 20% were using an effective method prior to the procedure, with 78% using an effective method afterward.

One issue in menstrual induction research is the likelihood of a woman being pregnant in her fifth week of menstrual delay as compared to the sixth and seventh weeks LMP. All such studies have concluded that the probability of pregnancy rises rapidly from the fifth to seventh week of menstrual delay, which is why the woman is advised to wait if at all possible until after her 35th or even 42nd day LMP. This is in no way to conclude that fifth-week procedures are unwarranted or unsafe for those in whom any other alternative would be impractical.

The IFRP found that twice as many women were pregnant if they were still amenorrheic in their sixth week rather than in the fifth week; another major review showed 54% proven pregnant in the fifth week LMP and 84% pregnant in the sixth week LMP. Some of these results can be affected by the accuracy of each operator's ability to evaluate uterine size and the effectiveness of the pregnancy testing procedures used. Nevertheless, it is clear that when faced with a delayed period, *only a few days* of amenorrhea can greatly change the probability of a woman being pregnant.

CONCLUSION

Menstrual induction and suction curettage are simple, safe, and effective methods of uterine aspiration. Although it is important for the provider to master the skills of physical examination, estimation of gestational age, dilation, sounding, aspiration and management of complications, the psychosocial aspects of pregnancy termination must always be remembered. Sensitive and thorough client counseling is at least as important in providing abortion services as are the technical aspects. The concept of "support" is probably more important in abortion counseling than in other family planning activities. If the provider can maintain an emotional foundation for the client from the moment of first contact through the period of postprocedure psychological healing, the abortion service will be truly therapeutic.

Selected Readings

American Public Health Association: Recommended program guide for abortion services (revised 1979). American Journal of Public Health 70(6): 652, June 1980

Andolsek L, Miller E, Bernard R: A comparison of flexible and nonflexible plastic cannulae for performing first trimester abortion. International Journal of Gynecology and Obstetrics 14(3): 199, 1976

Anonymous: The resumption of menstrual cycles after abortion. Research in Reproduction 10(2): 1, March 1978

Anonymous: Methods, weeks of gestation key in abortion complications. Contraceptive Technology Update 1(7): 96, October 1980

Anonymous: Common complications in first trimester abortions. Contraceptive Technology Update 2(1): 4, January 1981

Anonymous: Choosing, using pregnancy tests. Contraceptive Technology Update 3(1): 7, January 1982

Asher JD: Abortion counseling. American Journal of Public Health 62(5): 686, May 1972

Bhatia S. Faruque ASG, Chakraborty J: Assessing menstrual regulation performed by paramedics in rural Bangladesh. Studies in Family Planning 11(6): 213, June 1980

Bhuiyan SN, Burkhart MC: Maternal and public health benefits of menstrual regulation in Chittagong. International Journal of Gynecology and Obstetrics 20(2): 105, 1982

Bracken MB, Klerman LV, Bracken M: Abortion, adoption or motherhood: An empirical study of decision-making during pregnancy. American Journal of Obstetrics and Gynecology 130(3): 251, February 1, 1978

Brewer C: Third time unlucky: A study of women who have three or more legal abortions. Journal of Biosocial Science 9: 99, January 1977

Burkman RT, Tonascia JA, Atienza MF, et al: Untreated endocervical gonorrhea and endometritis following elective abortion. American Journal of Obstetrics and Gynecology 126(6): 648, November 15, 1976

Burnhill MS, Armstead JW: Reducing the morbidity of vacuum aspiration abortion. International Journal of Gynecology and Obstetrics 16(3): 204, 1978

Burnhill MS, Edelman DA, Armstead JW: The relationship between gestational age and the weight of the products of conception. Advances in Planned Parenthood 13(3/4): 9, 1978

Cates W: Adolescent abortions in the United States. Journal of Adolescent Health Care 1(1): 18, September 1980

Cates W: "Abortion myths and realities": Who is misleading whom? American Journal of Obstetrics and Gynecology 142(8): 954, April 15, 1982

Cates W. Grimes DA, Smith JC: Abortion as a treatment for unwanted pregnancy: The number two sexually-transmitted condition. Advances in Planned Parenthood 12(3): 115, 1978

Cates W, Hogue CR, Tietze C: Repeat induced abortions: Do they affect future childbearing? Fertility and Sterility 35(2): 236, February 1981 (abstract)

Cates W, Rochat RW, Grimes DA, et al: Legalized abortion: Effect on national trends of maternal and abortion-related mortality (1940 through 1976). American Journal of Obstetrics and Gynecology 132(2): 211, September 15, 1978

Cates W, Schultz KF, Grimes DA: Dilatation and evacuation for induced abortion in developing countries: advantages and disadvantages. Studies in Family Planning 11(4): 128, April 1980

Cates W, Smith JC, Rochat RW, et al: Mortality from abortion and childbirth: Are the statistics biased? Journal of the American Medical Association 248(2): 192, July 9, 1982

Chi I, Miller ER, Fortney J, et al: A study of abortion in countries where abortions are legally restricted. Journal of Reproductive Medicine 18(1): 15, January 1977

Cook RJ, Dickens BM: A decade of international change in abortion law: 1967–1977. American Journal of Public Health 68(7): 637, July 1978

Cutler JC: The risk of abortion denied, in Holtrop HR, Waife RS, Bustamante W, et al: New Developments in Fertility Regulation. Chestnut Hill, MA, The Pathfinder Fund, 1976, p 109

Daling JR, Emanuel I: Induced abortion and subsequent outcome of pregnancy in a series of American women. New England Journal of Medicine 297(23): 1241, December 9, 1977

Daling JR, Spadoni LR, Emanuel I: Role of induced abortion in secondary infertility. Obstetrics and Gynecology 57(1): 59, January 1981

David HP, Friedman HL, van der Tak J, et al (eds): Abortion in Psychosocial Perspective: Trends in Transnational Research. New York, Springer, 1978, 334 pp

DeCherney AH, Romero R, Naftolin F: Surgical management of unruptured ectopic pregnancy. Fertility and Sterility 35(1): 21, January 1981

Edelman DA, Brenner WE, Berger GS: The effectiveness and complications of abortion by dilation and vacuum aspiration versus dilation and rigid curettage. American Journal of Obstetrics and Gynecology 119(4): 473, June 15, 1974

Falk JR: Counseling the patient before menstrual induction, in Holtrop HR, Waife RS, Bustamante W, et al (ed): New Developments in Fertility Regulation. Chestnut Hill, MA, The Pathfinder Fund, 1976, p 201

Fielding WC, Lee S, Friedman EA: Continued pregnancy after failed first trimester abortion. Obstetrics and Gynecology 52(1): 56, July 1978

Fielding WL, Sachtleben MR, Friedman LM, et al: Comparison of women seeking early and late abortion. American Journal of Obstetrics and Gynecology 131(3): 304, June 1, 1978

Fortney JA, Laufe LE: Menstrual regulation—risks and benefits, in Sciarra JJ, Zatuchni GI, Speidel JJ (eds): Risks and Benefits and Controversies in Fertility Control. Hagertown, MD, Harper and Row, 1978, p 274

Fortney JA, Vengadasalam, D: Disposable menstrual regulation kits in a non-throw-away economy. Contraception 21(3): 235, March 1980

Freiman SM, Wulff GJL: Management of uterine perforation following elective abortion. Obstetrics and Gynecology 50(6): 647, December 1977

Fylling P, Jerve F: Contraceptive practice before and after termination of pregnancy. Contraception 15(3): 347, March 1977

Gallen ME, Narkavonkit T, Tomaro JB, et al: Traditional Abortion Practices. Research Triangle Park, NC, International Fertility Research Program, 1981, 100 pp

Golditch IM, Glasser MH: The use of laminaria tents for cervical dilation prior to vacuum aspiration abortion. American Journal of Obstetrics and Gynecology 119(4): 481, June 15, 1974

Goldsmith A: Intrauterine devices in the immediate postabortal period, in Holtrop HR, Waife RS, Bustamante W, et al (eds): New Developments in Fertility Regulation. Chestnut Hill, MA, The Pathfinder Fund, 1976, p 182

Goldsmith A, Edelman DA, Brenner WE: Contraception immediately after abortion. Advances in Planned Parenthood 9(3/4): 38, 1975

Grimes DA: Pregnancy persists despite abortion. Contraceptive Technology Update 1(8): 118, November 1980

Grimes DA, Cates W: Deaths from paracervical anesthesia used for first trimester abortion, 1972–1975. New England Journal of Medicine 295(25): 1397, December 16, 1976

Grimes DA, Cates W: Complications from legally-induced abortion: A review. Obstetrical and Gynecological Survey 34(3): 177, March 1979

Grimes DA, Cates W, Tyler CW: Comparative risk of death from legally induced abortion in hospitals and nonhospital facilities. Obstetrics and Gynecology 51(3): 323, March 1978

Grimes DA, Schulz KF, Cates W, et al: Midtrimester abortion by dilation and evacuation: A safe and practical alternative. New England Journal of Medicine 296(20): 1141, May 19, 1977

de Hamilton GM: Social implications of unwanted pregnancy, in Holtrop HR, Waife RS, Bustamante W, et al (eds): New Developments in Fertility Regulation. Chestnut Hill, MA, The Pathfinder Fund, 1976, p 133

Harlap S, Shiono PH: Alcohol, smoking and incidence of spontaneous abortions in the first and second trimester. Lancet 2: 173, July 26, 1980

Harlap S, Shiono PH, Ramcharan S, et al: A prospective study of spontaneous fetal losses after induced abortions. New England Journal of Medicine 301(13): 677, September 27, 1979

Hazekamp JT: Ectopic pregnancy: Diagnostic dilemma and delay. International Journal of Gynecology and Obstetrics 17(6): 598, 1980

Henshaw SK, Forrest JD, Sullivan E, et al: Abortion services in the United States, 1979 and 1980. Family Planning Perspectives 14(1): 5, January/February 1982

Hensleigh PA, Leslie W, Dixon E, et al: Reduced dose of Rh(D) immune globulin following induced first-trimester abortion. American Journal of Obsterics and Gynecology 129(4): 413, October 15, 1977

Hern WM, Andrikopoulos b (eds): Abortion in the Seventies. New York, National Abortion Federation, 1977, 296 pp

Hern WM, Corrigan B: What about us? Staff reactions to D&E. Advances in Planned Parenthood 15(1): 3, 1980

Hodgson JE: Major complications of 20,248 consecutive first trimester abortions: problems of fragmented care. Advances in Planned Parenthood 9(3/4): 52, 1975

Holtrop HR, Waife RS, Bustamante W, et al (eds): New Developments in Fertility Regulation. Chestnut Hill, MA, The Pathfinder Fund, 1976, 266 pp

Hogue CJR: An evaluation of studies concerning reproduction after first trimester induced abortion. International Journal of Gynecology and Obstetrics 15(2): 167, 1977

Hughes GJ: The early diagnosis of ectopic pregnancy. British Journal of Surgery 66: 789, 1979

Hunt WB: Pregnancy tests: The current status. Population Reports J(7), Washington, DC, George Washington University, November 1975

Isaacs JH, Wilhoite RW: Aspiration cytology of the endometrium: Office and hospital sampling procedures. American Journal of Obstetrics and Gynecology 118(5): 679, March 1, 1974

Jerome M, Armstead J, Burnhill MS, et al: Early recognition of ectopic pregnancy at a free-standing abortion clinic. Advances in Planned Parenthood 15(4): 144, 1981

Jones JE: The counselor and the physician: The preterm experience. Advances in Planned Parenthood 8: 196, 1973

Karman H: The paramedic abortionist. Clinical Obstetrics and Gynecology 15: 379, June 1972

Karman H, Potts M: Very early abortion using syringe as a vacuum source. Lancet 1: 1051, May 13, 1972

Keith L, et al: Monitoring care in abortion clinics. Journal of Reproductive Medicine 21(3): 163, September 1978

Kelly HA: Curettage without anesthesia on the office table. American Journal of Obstetrics and Gynecology 9: 78, 1925

Kerenyi TD, Glscock EL, Horowitz ML: Reasons for delayed abortion: Results of 400 interviews. American Journal of Obstetrics and Gynecology 117(3): 299, October 1, 1973

Kessel E: Estimated incidence of pregnancy by duration of amenorrhea. Advances in Planned Parenthood 9(3/4): 16, 1975

Kessel E, Brenner WE, Stathes GH: Menstrual regulation in family planning services. American Journal of Public Health 65(7): 731, July 1975

Koetsawang S, Saha A, Pachauri S: Study of "spontaneous" abortion in Thailand. International Journal of Gynecology and Obstetrics 15(5): 361, 1978

Ladipo OA, Ojo OA, James S, et al: Menstrual regulation in Ibadan, Nigeria. International Journal of Gynecology and Obstetrics 15(5): 428, 1978

Lahteenmaki P, Ylostalo P, Sipinen S, et al: Return of ovulation after abortion and after discontinuation of oral contraceptives. Fertility and Sterility 34(3): 246, September 1980

Lampe LG, Batar I, Bernard RP, et al: Effects of smoking and induced abortion on pregnancy outcome. IPPF Medical Bulletin 15(2): 3, April 1981

Laufe LE: The menstrual regulation procedure. Studies in Family Planning 8(10): 253, October 1977

LeBolt SA, Grimes DA, Cates W: Mortality from abortion and childbirth: Are the populations comparable? Journal of the American Medical Association 248(2): 188, July 9, 1982

Lee LT, Paxman JM: Legal aspects of menstrual regulation. Studies in Family Planning 8(10): 273, October 1977

Levin AA, Schoenbaum SC, Monson RR, et al: Association of induced abortion with subsequent pregnancy loss. Journal of the American Medical Association 243(24): 2495, June 27, 1980

Levin AA, Schoenbaum SC, Stubblefield PG, et al: Ectopic pregnancy and prior induced abortion. American Journal of Public Health 72(3): 253, March 1982

Lilaram D, Basu S, Khan PK, et al: Evaluation of 496 menstrual regulation and abortion patients in Calcutta. International Journal of Gynecology and Obstetrics 15(6): 503, 1978

Liskin LS: Complications of abortion in developing countries. Population Reports F(7), Baltimore, Population Information Program, July 1980, 50 pp

Lyon FA: Ectopic pregnancy as a complication of elective first trimester abortion. Advances in Planned Parenthood 10(4): 244, 1975

Madore C, Hawes WE, Many F, et al: A study on the effects of induced abortion on subsequent pregnancy outcome. American Journal of Obstetrics and Gynecology 139(5): 516, March 1, 1981

Marshall BR: Emergency room vacuum curettage for incomplete abortion. Journal of Reproductive Medicine 6(4): 61, April 1971

McElin TW, Giese TM: Complication of abortion performed with a plastic suction curet: Intrauterine loss of the curet tip. American Journal of Obstetrics and Gynecology 132(3): 343, October 1, 1978

Measham AR, Obaidullah M, Rosenberg MJ et al: Complications from induced abortion in Bangladesh related to types of practitioner and methods, and impact on mortality. Lancet 1: 199, January 24, 1981

Miller ER, Fortnery JA, Kessel E: Early vacuum aspiration: Minimizing procedures to nonpregnant women. Family Planning Perspective 8(1): 33, January/February 1976

Miller E, McFarland V, Burnhill MS, et al: Impact of the abortion experience on contraception acceptance. Advances in Planned Parenthood 12(1): 15, 1977

Miller ER, Wood JL, Andolsek L, et al: First trimester abortion by vacuum aspiration: Interphysician variability. International Journal of Gynecology and Obstetrics 16(2): 144, 1978

Moberg PJ: Uterine perforation in connection with vacuum aspiration for legal abortion. International Journal of Gynecology and Obstetrics 14(1): 77, 1976

Newman L, Murphy M: Menstrual induction: II. Psycho-social aspects. Advances in Planned Parenthood 9: 11, 1973

Obel EB: Risk of spontaneous abortion following legally induced abortion. Acta Obstetricia et Gynecologica Scandinavica 59: 131, 1980

Okojie SE: Induced illegal abortions in Benin City, Nigeria. International Journal of Gynecology and Obstetrics 14(6): 517, 1976

Oronsaye AU: The outcome of pregnancies subsequent to induced and spontaneous abortion. International Journal of Gynecology and Obstetrics 17(3): 274, 1979

Ott ER: Cervical dilation: A review. Population Report F(6), Washington, DC, George Washington University, September 1977

Pan American Health Organization: Epidemiology of abortion and practices of fertility regulation in Latin America: Selected reports. PAHO Scientific Publication Number 306, Washington, DC, PAHO, 1975, 142 pp

Peterson HB, Grimes DA, Cates W. et al: Comparative risk of death from induced abortion at less than 12 weeks' gestation performed with local versus general anesthesia. American Journal of Obstetrics and Gynecology 141(7): 763, December 1, 1981

Potts M, Diggory P, Peel J: Abortion. Cambridge, Cambridge University Press, 1977, 575 pp

Powe CE, McGee JA: Combined outpatient laparoscopic sterilization with therapeutic abortion. American Journal of Obstetrics and Gynecology 126(5): 565, November 1, 1976

Rosenthal MB, Rothchild E: Some psychological considerations in adolescent pregnancy and abortion. Advances in Planned Parenthood 9(3/4): 60, 1975

Rubin GL, Cates W, Gold J, et al: Fetal ectopic pregnancy after attempted legally induced abortion. Journal of the American Medical Association 244(15): 1705, October 10, 1980

Rushwan H: Epidemiological analysis and reproductive characteristics of incomplete abortion patients in Khartoum, in Gerais AS, Rushwan H (eds): Proceedings of the Seminar on Recent Advances in Family Planning Technology. Khartoum, Sudan Fertility Control Association, 1977

Rushwan H, Doodoh A, Chi I, et al: Contraceptive practice after women have undergone "spontaneous" abortion in Indonesia and Sudan. International Journal of Gynecology and Obstetrics 15(3): 241, 1977

Rushwan HE, Ferguson JG, Bernard RP: Hospital counseling in Khartoum: A study of factors affecting contraceptive acceptance after abortion. International Journal of Gynecology and Obstetrics 15(5): 440, 1978

Safilos-Rothchild C: Why some women prefer abortion to contraception. Contemporary Obstetrics and Gynecology 4: 125, October 1974

Sambhi JS: Abortion by massage—"bomoh." IPPF Medical Bulletin 11(1): 3, February 1977

Schneider SM, Thompson DS: Repeat aborters. American Journal of Obstetrtics and Gynecology 126(3): October 1, 1976

Schoenbaum SC, Monson RR, Stubblefield PG, et al: Outcome of the delivery following an induced or spontaneous abortion. American Journal of Obstetrics and Gynecology 136(1): 19, January 1, 1980

Sciarra JJ, Zatuchni GI, Spidel JJ (eds): Risks Benefits and Controversies in Fertility Control. Hagerstown, MD, Harper and Row, 1978, 601 pp

Scotti RJ, Karman HL: Menstrual regulation and early pregnancy termination performed by paraprofessionals under medical supervision. Contraception 14(4): 367, October 1976

Selik RM, Cates W, Tyler CW: Behavioral factors contributing to abortion deaths: A new approach to mortality studies. Obstetrics and Gynecology 58(5): 631, November 1981

Simpson JY: Clinical Lectures of the Diseases of Women. Edinburgh, R Clark, 1872, 789 pp

Smith GM, Stubblefield PG, Chirchirillo L, et al: Pain of first-trimester abortion: Its quantification and relations with other variables. American Journal of Obstetrics and Gynecology 133(5): 489, March 1, 1979

Smith R, Gardner RW, Steinhoff P, et al: The effect of induced abortion on the incidence of Down's syndrome in Hawaii. Family Planning Perspectives 12(4): 201, July/August 1980

Smith RG, Palmore JA, Steinhoff PG: The potential reduction of medical complications from induced abortion. International Journal of Gynecology and Obstetrics 15(4): 337, 1978

Sonne-holm S, Heisterberg L, Hebjorn S, et al: Prophylactic antibiotics in first-trimester abortions: A clinical, controlled trial. American Journal of Obstetrics and Gynecology 139(6): 693, March 15, 1981

Spence MR, King TM, Brockman M: The cold sterilization of abortion cannulae. International Journal of Gynecology and Obstetrics 15(4): 369, 1978

Stewart FH, Burnhill MS, Bozorgi N: Reduced dose of Rh immunoglobulin following first trimester pregnancy termination. Obstetrics and Gynecology 51(3): 318, March 1978

Swigar ME, Breslin R, Pouzzner MG, et al: Interview follow-up of abortion applicant dropouts. Social Psychiatry 11: 135, 1976

Tietze C: The effect of legalization of abortion on population growth and public health. Family Planning Perspectives 7(3): 123, May/June 1975

Tietze C: Comparative morbidity and mortality in abortion and contraception, in Hern WM, Andrikopoulos B (eds): Abortion in the Seventies. New York, National Abortion Federation, 1977, p 57

Tietze C: Induced Abortion: A World Review, 1981. New York, The Population Council, 1981, 113 pp

Tyrer L: Postabortal use of oral contraceptives, in Holtrop HR, Waife RS, Bustamante W, et al (eds): New Development in Fertility Regulation. Chestnut Hill, MA, The Pathfinder Fund, 1976, p 177

Valle RF, Sabbagha RE: Management of first trimester pregnancy failures. Obstetrics and Gynecology 55(5): 625, May 1980

Van der Vlugt, P: Uterine aspiration techniques. Population Report F(3), Washington, DC, George Washington University, June 1973

Van der Vlugt, P: Menstrual regulation update. Population Report F(4), Washington, DC, George Washington University, May 1974

Varner M, deProsse CA, Digre K: Ectopic pregnancy and first-trimester pregnancy termination. Advances in Planned Parenthood 15(2): 64, 1980

Waife RS: Traditional methods of birth control in Zaire. Pathpapers number 4. Chestnut Hill, MA, The Pathfinder Fund, December 1978, 18 pp

World Health Organization: Gestation, birthweight and spontaneous abortion in pregnancy after induced abortion. Lancet 1: 142, January 20, 1979

Wulff GJL, Freiman SM: Elective abortion: Complications seen in a free-standing clinic. Obstetrics and gynecology 49(3): 351, March 1977

Zatuchni GI, Sciarra JJ, Spiedel JJ: Pregnancy Termination: Procedures, Safety and New Developments. Hagerstown, MD, Harper and Row, 1979, 447 pp

Referral for Sterilization

6

Millions of couples are choosing sterilization as their means of contraception; sterilization procedures are among the most frequently performed surgical operations in the world. During the 1970s the number of people sterilized increased from 20 million to 100 million. In the United States, more couples prevent unwanted pregnancy through voluntary sterilization than any other single method of family planning. Health providers who are counseling their clients about family planning will therefore be asked about sterilization frequently. This chapter is not intended to teach the provider how to perform sterilization, but rather to prepare the provider for counseling and referring the client who chooses this method of family planning.

The essence of voluntary sterilization to be communicated in the counseling session is twofold—*permanence* and *effectiveness*. Despite the progress being made in the sophisticated techniques of reversal (see pages 242 and 247), sterilization should generally be discussed as an irrevocable decision to end reproductive capacity. The great advantage of sterilization is its unsurpassed effectiveness in preventing pregnancy—over 99% for both male and female sterilization. There is little wonder why voluntary sterilization is so popular for those couples who have completed their childbearing.

Voluntary sterilization occupies a logical end point in the time span of a couple's reproductive planning. Adolescents and young couples—married or unmarried—tend to use contraception for *preventing* a first pregnancy and will therefore use highly effective methods such as oral contraceptives, or condoms with foam.

Couples who are having children purposefully then face the challenge of *spacing* pregnancies, when the pill or IUD, or less effective but safer methods such as the diaphragm, are ideal. The dilemma facing couples who have completed their desired family size is how to prevent unwanted pregnancy over the *many remaining years* of reproductive capacity. For these couples, intrauterine devices (IUDs) are an excellent *reversible* choice and sterilization an excellent *permanent* choice.

The decision to choose sterilization must be preceded by a discussion of the complete range of contraceptive alternatives (see Chapter 1) under circumstances that allow for a truly informed and free choice. But first, of course, the counselor must fully understand what these procedures involve. This chapter describes the surgical techniques for female and male sterilization, possible side-effects and complications, and prospects for reversibility. The counseling session for sterilization is then discussed—the topics to include and the client questions that can be expected.

FEMALE STERILIZATION

The practice of sterilization solely for voluntary permanent contraception is primarily a 20th century phenomenon. In the past such operations were performed only for therapeutic medical indications. The growth of voluntary sterilization began very slowly and was limited by restrictive institutional and professional policies and attitudes. Until 1969, for instance, the American College of Obstetrics and Gynecology recommended that voluntary sterilization be performed only if the woman met certain guidelines of age and number of living children, such as being 30 years old with four children. Today the profession recognizes that voluntary sterilization is an individual choice regardless of the number of children a woman may or may not have. Sterilization should be routinely performed on request when the physician is satisfied that the woman is basing her decision on adequate information and awareness of her contraceptive choices.

Terminology: Approach and Occlusion

The many different terms used to describe the various surgical techniques for female sterilization can often lead to a confusing impression. It is best to simplify the discussion by thinking of each

Table 6-1. Female Sterilization Terminology.	
Approaches through the *abdomen*: Laparoscopy* Minilaparotomy Laparotomy **Approaches through the *vaginal cul-de-sac*:** Culdoscopy* Colpotomy	**Methods of *occlusion*:** Tubal ligation Silastic ring Plastic clip Electrocoagulation Removal of tubes, ovaries, uterus (-ectomy)
*Endoscopic.	

technique consisting of two parts—the approach and the method of tubal occlusion (blockage, interruption).

Approach. The surgeon can approach the fallopian tubes from one of two directions—through the abdomen or through the vaginal cul-de-sac (Table 6-1 and Figure 6-1). The abdominal approach is the most common and is used by the two techniques that are described in detail here (laparoscopy and minilaparotomy). The abdominal approach is also used in regular laparotomy. Colpotomy and culdoscopy are the two techniques that use the vaginal approach, but because of their limited use, we do not discuss them further in this chapter.

Each approach is further subdivided as to whether an endoscope is used. An endoscope, used in many medical applications, is a tubular instrument containing optical lenses and a source of light to permit viewing of internal organs. The endoscope used in laparos-

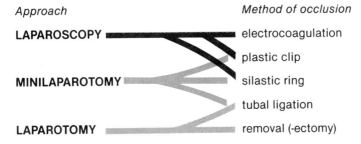

Figure 6-1. *Sterilization approaches discussed in this chapter, showing occlusion options usually available.*

copy is called a *laparoscope* (Figure 6-2). It enables the surgeon to use a very small incision and to occlude the fallopian tubes without bringing them outside the abdomen. The other abdominal methods of female sterilization are performed by bringing the fallopian tubes through a wider incision for occlusion.

Occlusion. There are various ways to occlude the fallopian tubes—to make them incapable of transporting the ovum and preventing the spermatozoa access. Rarely, the entire tube, ovary, and/or uterus can be removed (salpingectomy, oophorectomy, and hysterectomy). Usually, the tubes are simply interrupted. The tubes can be tied and cut (ligation), the tubes can be electrically burned (electrocoagulation), a knuckle of each tube can be trapped inside a tight silastic ring, or the tubes can be clamped shut with a plastic clip. Most of these methods of occlusion could be used with all the approaches listed above. When one hears a term such as "laparoscopy," therefore, although it clearly defines the *approach* used, it does not automatically indicate which method of occlusion is used.

This chapter focuses on the two methods of elective female sterilization most widely used in the world today—laparoscopy and minilaparotomy. Both use the abdominal approach through small incisions. In laparoscopy an endoscope is used; in minilaparotomy the tubes are pulled through the incision and occluded under direct visualization. A comparison of their techniques, requirements, and effects is presented below.

Laparoscopy

Laparoscopy is becoming the most common approach to female sterilization in the United States today. Although it requires sophisticated equipment, the surgical technique for laparoscopy is relatively simple and enables the procedure to be accomplished on an

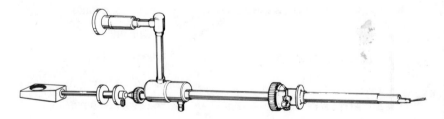

Figure 6-2. *The laparoscope.*

outpatient basis. This eliminates the costly hospitalization required for the traditional methods of postpartum and interval laparotomy. Laparoscopy still must be performed in a sophisticated medical setting, however, so that a wider abdominal incision and more extensive surgery can be performed if necessary.

The laparoscope.   The laparoscope is a stainless steel instrument 7–12 cm in diameter. It contains several channels, depending on its design: one channel has lenses for visualizing the abdominal contents, one channel carries the high intensity pinpoint light source, and sometimes there is a channel through which operating instruments can be inserted. The laparoscope is inserted into the abdomen through a metal sleeve.

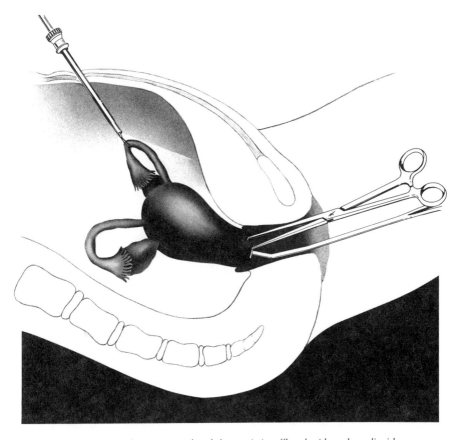

Figure 6-3.   *In laparoscopy the abdomen is insufflated with carbon dioxide.*

Technique. In order to make room for the laparoscope to manuever inside the abdomen, the abdominal cavity is first filled with a gas (insufflation), usually CO_2, through a needle until the abdomen is taut. The patient is then placed in the Trendelenburg position (head lower than the feet) so that the bowel falls away from the pelvis and the reproductive organs can be easily visualized.

Just below the navel, a 1.5–2-cm (½-in.) incision is made through the skin. The sleeve for the laparoscope with a trocar (sharp pointed instrument) inside is then inserted through the peritoneum. The trocar is removed and replaced with a laparoscope.

A uterine elevator (similar to a uterine sound), which has been introduced through the cervix and into the uterine cavity, is used to manipulate the uterus as necessary to bring it and the fallopian tubes within sight of the laparoscope (Figure 6-3). In those circumstances when the surgeon is using a *two-incision* technique, a sleeve for the grasping forceps is introduced into the abdominal cavity through a separate incision. Otherwise the forceps are used through the laparoscope itself.

When the tubes are identified, each tube in turn is grasped with the forceps approximately 2 cm from the uterus. At this point either a silastic ring (also called a *Yoon band* or *Falope ring*) is slipped over a "knuckle" of the tube (Figure 6-4), or a plastic clip is applied (Figure 6-5). The ring and clip are so tight that the inside of the tube is squeezed shut. Alternatively, by applying an electric current through the forceps, the surgeon can electrocoagulate a portion of the tube, and the tube will be sealed with scar tissue. Electrocoagulation is associated with a slightly higher incidence of complications, including bowel burns. Since the silastic ring or clip apparently destroys a smaller portion of the tube, the small chance for reversing the sterilization is theoretically higher with use of these occlusion methods (see page 242). After tubal occlusion, the laparoscope is removed and the incision closed. The entire procedure averages about 20 minutes.

The patient will generally be asked to report to the facility in the morning and can expect to be discharged within several hours, assuming a normal recovery. She may experience discomfort for a day or two as a result of the gas insufflation. Normal activities can be resumed the next day, but the patient should refrain from sexual intercourse or douching for 3 weeks. If nonabsorbable sutures or clips were used to close the incision, the woman will have to return in a week for their removal. Other follow-up visits may be scheduled.

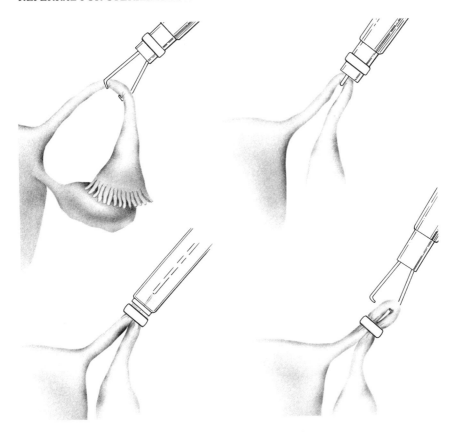

Figure 6-4. *Tubal occlusion using the silastic ring.*

One risk of laparoscopy comes from the "blind" insertion of the insufflation needle and sharp trocar into the abdomen—it is possible to pierce the aorta or other major vessel, or the bowels, although this is extremely rare with use of the proper technique. So-called open laparoscopy has been proposed to avoid this risk. In this technique, a narrow opening is made in the peritoneum under direct vision as in normal laparotomy. A specially designed sleeve is used

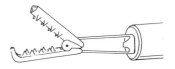

Figure 6-5. *The plastic clip.*

for introducing the laparoscope into the abdomen. Laparoscopy is then performed as usual. This method avoids the dangers of sharp trocar insertion; however, the instrumentation required is still complex and expensive.

Anesthesia.   Laparoscopy can be safely performed using a local anesthesia such as lidocaine, with preoperative medication such as a combination of intravenous meperidine (Demerol) and diazepam (Valium). Because of transient pain when electrocoagulation is used, the surgeon may choose to apply a topical anesthetic to the tubes. Many surgeons still use general anesthesia for laparoscopy; general anesthesia will keep the patient still and will also keep the abdomen more relaxed. However, this practice is usually unnecessary except when medically indicated. The use of general anesthesia significantly heightens the patient's risk of complications—one recent estimate put the increased mortality risk at five times that when using local anesthesia for laparoscopy.

Contraindications.   A woman should not undergo laparoscopy if she has cardiorespiratory insufficiency, because the gas insufflation and operative position will be a dangerous strain. Certain physical conditions will require a larger abdominal incision, making traditional laparotomy a more appropriate approach. These conditions include extreme obesity, previous lower abdominal surgery, and prior pelvic inflammation with known adhesions (Table 6-2). As with all surgery, the presence of various illnesses will preclude the procedure being performed on an outpatient basis. If a client is known to have a contraindication to laparoscopy, other sterilization and contraceptive alternatives should be presented to her.

Effectiveness and safety.   The effectiveness in preventing pregnancy for all methods of tubal occlusion performed by laparoscopy is over 99%. Occlusion by electrocoagulation seems to be slightly more effective; occlusion by the ring or clip is slightly less effective,

| Table 6-2. |
| Contraindications to Outpatient Laparoscopy. |
| • Cardiorespiratory insufficiency
• Excessive obesity
• Pelvic pathology, especially adhesions
• Serious illness |

Table 6-3.
Laparoscopy Complications.
• Bleeding • Uterine perforation • Accidental burns • Bowel trauma • Major vessel perforation

but these variations range from 1 to 7 per 1000 sterilizations and are not clinically significant. It has been recently estimated by the U.S. Centers for Disease Control (CDC) that half of all sterilization "failures" in the United States are due to the woman being pregnant (and undiagnosed) at the time of the procedure.

Most estimates for the frequency of complications due to laparoscopy range below 4% (Table 6-3). These complications included bleeding, uterine perforation, accidental burns, and bowel trauma. Each of these complications occurs in less than 1% of all procedures. Complications occur slightly more frequently with electrocoagulation, and accidental burns can be serious. Major vessel injury resulting from improper insertion of the insufflation needle or trocar occur at a rate of 9 per 10,000 procedures, according to a British study.

What is particularly reassuring is the near total absence of infection as a result of laparoscopic sterilization, in marked contrast to other sterilization methods, especially those using the vaginal approach. The rare laparoscopy complications usually occur when the surgeon is actually performing the procedure or during the immediate recovery period. Thus, they can be managed while the patient is still in the medical facility.

There is disagreement among researchers about the effects of sterilization on subsequent menstrual function. A "poststerilization syndrome" has been described in some woman that includes increased menstrual pain and irregular bleeding patterns. However, preliminary studies by the CDC and the International Fertility Research Program (IFRP) have found that after sterilization, the number of days of menstruation, the amount the flow and the frequency of intermenstrual spotting all were unchanged. Menstrual pattern changes after sterilization appear to be frequently associated with the discontinuation of oral contraceptive or IUD use at the time of the procedure.

Table 6-4. Comparative Mortality Rates.	
	Deaths*
Laparoscopy	3–10
Minilaparotomy	8
Laparotomy	10–25
Vasectomy	1
Maternity	
Developed countries	65
Developing countries	up to 700

Adapted from IPAVS, 1981, Peterson et al, 1981, and others.
*Deaths per 100,000 procedures or live births.

Female sterilization, like other contraceptive use, lowers the cumulative lifetime risk of the woman experiencing an ectopic (tubal) pregnancy. But in the rare instance when a woman who has been sterilized becomes pregnant anyway, she will run a significantly greater risk that the pregnancy will be ectopic—somewhere between 5% and 20%, compared to the normal risk of 0.5%. But since pregnancy so rarely occurs after sterilization, the overall risk of a subsequent ectopic pregnancy among women undergoing sterilization is less than 2 per 1000 procedures. Apparently it is more likely for a pregnancy to be ectopic after the first poststerilization year. Ectopic pregnancy is more likely to occur when the tubes are occluded by electrocoagulation than by other methods and are especially likely after sterilization reversal is attempted.

Mortality resulting from laparoscopic sterilization is very low—current estimates range from 3 to 10 per 100,000 procedures (Table 6-4). As is common with a surgical procedure, this mortality risk is higher than that for the nonsurgical contraceptive alternatives such as the IUD or oral contraceptives (in young nonsmokers). For older women who smoke, the mortality risk from sterilization is lower than that for the pill (see page 55). All these rates compare very favorably to the mortality risk from pregnancy, which can range up to 700 per 100,000 live births in some developing countries.

Training and equipment. The major disadvantage of laparoscopic sterilization is that it requires sophisticated equipment that is expensive and prone to breakdowns. This equipment costs approximately 10 times that of the equipment for minilaparotomy, about U.S. $4500 in 1980. The equipment requires a highly trained gynecological surgeon to operate it and skilled technicians to maintain it. Since the effectiveness and safety of laparoscopy is at least matched by minilaparotomy (see below), "minilap" seems to be the preferable female sterilization procedure, especially in areas with limited resources for training laparoscopists and for equipment purchase and maintenance.

Minilaparotomy

Minilaparotomy ("minilap") simply means entering the abdomen through a small incision. It has become increasingly popular since the mid-1970s. Minilap requires only the simplest of surgical equipment and facilities and no special endoscopic training. Insufflation is unnecessary, eliminating this source of postoperative discomfort for the patient. Minilap is performed on an outpatient basis with local anesthesia, so that complication risks and inconvenience are minimized. It should also be less expensive. All methods of tubal occlusion can be used with minilap with effectiveness equal to laparoscopy.

Technique. Minilaparotomy depends on the use of a uterine elevator—an instrument similar to a uterine sound that is inserted into the uterine cavity through the cervix. The elevator is used to lift the uterus up close to the abdominal wall. This enables the operator to pinpoint the location of the small incision (less than 3 cm), just above the pubis (Figure 6-6A). As the uterus is lifted, so are the fallopian tubes. Using the uterine elevator to gently turn the uterus, the surgeon identifies each tube, pulls it through the incision (Figure 6-6B), and occludes it. The incision is then closed and the uterine elevator removed.

Occlusion can be accomplished either with the bands or clips described above, or by ligation (tying and cutting). There are several methods of ligation, the most common of which is called the *Pomeroy method.* A knuckle of the midportion of the fallopian tube is tied with absorbable catgut. The knuckle is then cut. After the suture is absorbed, the cut ends of the tube will fall away from each other and the openings eventually will be covered by peritoneal tissue

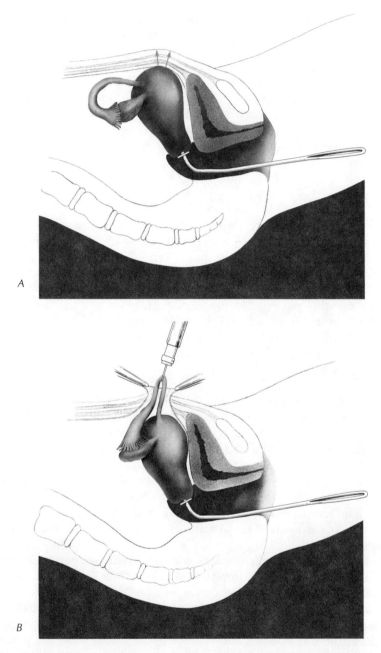

Figure 6-6. *Minilaparotomy. (A) The uterus is elevated to the abdominal wall by use of a uterine elevator. (B) Tubal ligation is accomplished through a small incision.*

Table 6-5. Contraindications to Outpatient Minilaparotomy.
• Extreme obesity • Pelvic pathology, especially adhesions • Serious illness

(abdominal lining). A simple instrument is used to apply the silastic band for minilap (the laparoscope is not necessary).

Minilaparotomy may take a little longer than laparoscopy to perform, but it is still usually completed within 20 minutes. Since the procedure is performed under local anesthesia, the patient's recovery time is short. As with laparoscopy, normal activities can be resumed the next day, but the patient should refrain from intercourse or douching for 3 weeks. If nonabsorbable sutures or clips were used to close the incision, the woman will have to return in a week for their removal. Other follow-up visits may be scheduled.

Anethesia. Minilaparotomy patients are usually given preoperative analgesia and sedation, such as a combination of intravenous meperidine (Demerol) and diazepam (Valium). Local anesthesia (such as lidocaine) at the incision site is sufficient, and general anesthesia is not necessary. Additional local anesthetic can be applied to the tubes themselves if the patient feels discomfort during occlusion.

Contraindications. The two major contraindications to performing sterilization by minilaparotomy are excessive obesity and pelvic pathology (Table 6-5). Excessive obesity will interfere with manipulation of the uterus and identification of the tubes and requires a larger incision. Pelvic pathology such as adhesions or rigid pelvic viscera will also prevent the uterus from being brought up to the incision site. As with laparoscopy, serious illness will preclude minilaparotomy from being performed on an outpatient basis.

Effectiveness and safety. Sterilization by minilap is as effective as any other approach—over 99%. As with laparoscopy, effectiveness varies slightly by method of occlusion, with ligation more effective than the ring.

Complications with minilap appear to be equivalent to those due to other approaches, occurring in about 3% of procedures (Table

Table 6-6. Minilaparotomy Complications.
• Bleeding • Uterine perforation • Bowel or bladder trauma

6-6). Minilap avoids the possibility of accidental burns from electro-coagulation or trauma from the trocar used in laparoscopy, but use of the uterine elevator adds a very small risk of uterine perforation. The surgeon will be able to manage uterine perforation safely (see pages 111 and 212 for more discussion of uterine perforation). The mortality rate for minilap sterilization has been estimated at 8 per 100,000 procedures (see Table 6-4).

Training and equipment. The hallmark of minilaparotomy is its simplicity. Well-trained abdominal surgeons can perform mini-lap without a background in endoscopy or insufflation. The operation can be performed in an outpatient clinic or any facility prepared for minor surgery, as long as specific contingency plans are in place for removing the patient to a hospital in case of rare complications. The equipment needed for minilap will be found in any surgical facility, since even the uterine elevator can be fashioned out of common instruments. Specially made elevators are also available.

Laparotomy

Before the development of laparoscopy and minilaparotomy, traditional laparotomy (abdominal surgery using a much larger incision) was the approach used for female sterilization. Laparotomy was and is most commonly used in the immediate postpartum period, within 48 hours after delivery. At this time the uterus is enlarged and relatively easy to reach through the incision without elevation. Occlusion is usually accomplished by Pomeroy ligation (Figure 6-7).

Postpartum. Postpartum laparotomy does not require special instruments and rarely adds to the length of the postpartum hospital stay. The procedure takes 20–30 minutes and can be performed under a wide variety of anesthetic techniques.

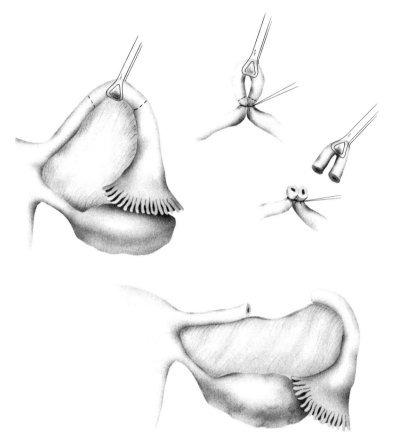

Figure 6-7. *Pomeroy ligation for interval laparotomy. A knuckle of the tube is grasped, ligated, and cut.*

Interval. Traditional laparotomy for sterilization not in the postpartum period ("interval" sterilization) is not commonly performed in most places today. It requires a 10-cm incision and general anethesia. The procedure requires a 3–5-day hospital stay and a lengthy postoperative recovery (4–6 weeks). Interval laparotomy may be necessary when the woman requesting sterilization has pelvic adhesions or other pathology, or if other surgical indications exist (removal of ovarian cysts, for example).

Effectiveness and safety. Sterilization by traditional laparotomy is as effective as other methods but has higher complication rates. Postoperative morbidity (principally infection or bleeding) occurs in 2%–4% of cases, and mortality has been estimated at 10–25 per 100,000 procedures (see Table 6-4).

Reversibility

As emphasized earlier, sterilization should be considered a choice for *permanent* contraception. It is true that much research and some progress is occurring in techniques for restoring the function of the occluded fallopian tubes. Nevertheless, these techniques require sophisticated and expensive microsurgical equipment, highly trained specialists, do not guarantee successful return to fertility, and carry risks of their own. The cost of a procedure to reverse female sterilization was about U.S. $5000 in 1980.

The motivations for couples seeking a reversal of sterilization are diverse. It has been estimated that two-thirds of reversal requests come from clients who have changed their marital status. But despite all the publicity about the issue of reversibility, the overall frequency of a reversal request is very low—probably about 1% of sterilizations performed. Furthermore, approximately only 20% of these requests will lead to an operation because various medical and physiological factors will contraindicate the reversal attempt (not the least of which is the amount of viable tube remaining). Thus reversal will be attempted only at a rate of about 2 per 1000 sterilization procedures.

Since premenopausal women who have undergone tubal occlusion are still ovulating, theoretically "all" that needs to be done to restore her ability to conceive is to reconnect the tubes. The surgical procedure that attempts this reconnection is called *reanastomosis*. Regardless of the method of occlusion that had been used, the surgeon must cut out the affected portion of the tube and attempt to put the ends back together, after making sure that the tubal openings are freed of the scar tissue that forms after sterilization.

Success rates. Specialists in sterilization reversal have reported success rates—defined as the patient carrying a viable pregnancy to term—ranging from 50% to 86%. The average time from the reversal operation to conception is about 10 months. The rate of pregnancy "wastage" (failure to deliver a live infant) is three times higher than normal in previously sterilized women (39% versus 13%).

Success in reversing sterilization is directly related to how much viable tube remains—something difficult to know for certain before opening the abdomen. Most surgeons agree that at least 3 cm of one tube must be viable to make the reversal attempt worthwhile. Electrocoagulation destroys several centimeters of tube and is the method of occlusion hardest to reverse. Pomeroy ligation and silastic bands are less destructive, and plastic clips theoretically should be the easiest to reverse.

Complications. The risk of ectopic (tubal) pregnancy developing in a woman after a sterilization reversal procedure is much higher than normal and is 10 times that in sterilized women who do not attempt reversal. Ectopic pregnancy is a potentially life-threatening condition (see pages 117 and 190 for more discussion of ectopic pregnancy). Additionally, because of the complexity of reversal operations, they are naturally performed under general anesthesia, with its attendant risks.

Despite these problems with current techniques for reversal of female sterilization, there is reason for optimism. Research into new methods of tubal sterilization continues and should result in the development of procedures that are much easier to reverse. Such an achievement would further improve the already remarkable popularity of voluntary sterilization for family planning.

MALE STERILIZATION

The male sterilization procedure is called *vasectomy,* which means cutting the *vas deferens* that carry spermatozoa from the testicles. Vasectomy is a much simpler and safer procedure than any female sterilization technique and yet is just as effective in preventing pregnancy. Since the 1950s it has rapidly gained popularity as a method of contraception and shares with the condom the distinction of being a direct male contribution to family planning.

Vasectomy's popularity, heavily influenced by cultural factors, varies greatly from country to country. In the United States it is estimated that one-half of all sterilization procedures performed are vasectomies. In India, Bangladesh, and Nepal, the proportion is over two-thirds. On the other hand, vasectomy is relatively rarely performed in most of Africa and Latin America.

Resistance to vasectomy among men in some countries or cultures may be assumed but is not necessarily impossible to overcome. In Thailand, for instance, 1975 data showed that only 2% of married men had chosen vasectomy—male sterilizations were performed one-tenth as often as female sterilizations. But one clinic at a Bangkok hospital surveyed their clients to discover some of the obstacles to vasectomy acceptance. By changing the hours the clinic was open, cutting down on waiting times, opening the clinic on weekends, providing transportation for clients, and making the clinic atmosphere more pleasant, the hospital was able in 3 years to triple the number of vasectomies performed there each month.

Vasectomy Technique

Technique. Vasectomy is performed on an outpatient basis (even in a provider's office) under local anesthesia. Each *vas deferens* is isolated by palpation, and an anesthetic (such as lidocaine) is injected at the incision site. The injection may cause some discomfort. Then a tiny incision (1 cm) is made in the scrotal sac for each vas. The vas is pulled through, ligated (tied), and cut (Figure 6-8). Sometimes the surgeon will use an electrocautery or, rarely, specially designed clips can be applied. The incisions are sutured, and the patient stays at the facility for a few hours before returning home.

The vasectomy patient should be able to resume normal activities the next day, although heavy manual labor is not recommended for several days. The surgeon may recommend that the patient wear an athletic supporter to ease postoperative discomfort in the scrotum. Vasectomy patients should expect some purple discoloration to develop at the incision site. Recommendations for the time to resume sexual intercourse range from 5 to 14 days after the procedure.

Contraindications. Contraindications to vasectomy are infrequent. They include genital or scrotal infection, bleeding disorders, or anticoagulant therapy (Table 6-7). The presence of a scrotal hernia, hydrocele (collection of fluid along the spermatic cord), variocele (varicose scrotal veins), undescended testicle (or history of this condition), or a thickened scrotum caused by filariasis (worms) make vasectomy more difficult to perform and usually dictate the use of general anethesia in a hospital setting. There are also psycho-

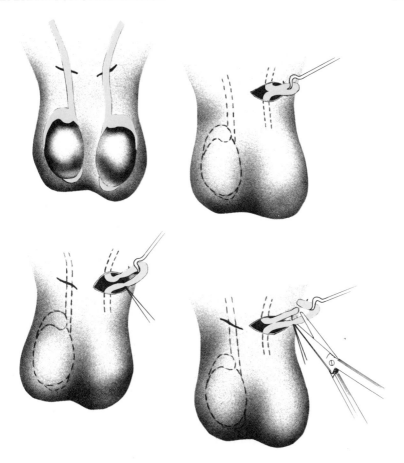

Figure 6-8. *Vasectomy. A small incision is made over each vas, and a knuckle of the vas is grasped, ligated, and cut.*

logical contraindications to vasectomy. For men with a history of impotence or other sexual dysfunction, vasectomy may intensify underlying psychological problems.

Effectiveness and safety. Vasectomy is as effective as female sterilization (99%), but its effect is *not* immediate. After the vas are tied, spermatozoa will remain in the seminal vesicles for some time, perhaps as long as 2 weeks or more. Condoms or other contraception should be used until the ejaculate is sperm-free. This determi-

Table 6-7. **Contraindications to Outpatient Vasectomy.**
• Genital or scrotal infection • Bleeding disorders and/or anticoagulant therapy • Scrotal hernia • Hydrocele or variocele • Undescended testicle • Thickened scrotum

nation must be made by laboratory examination, and it is prudent to obtain two consecutive sperm-free samples before confirming that the vasectomy has been effective. If the man cannot or will not return for these tests, a rule of thumb can be used that at least 20 ejaculations and a period of 3 weeks are necessary to clear the system of spermatozoa.

The overall complication rate for vasectomy is very low, about 3% or less. Complications include bleeding, infection, and hematoma (a collection of blood at the incision site) (Table 6-8). Hematoma may require surgical drainage. A granuloma (a tumorlike mass caused by inflammation) may form from reactions to the suture or leakage of sperm. Usually a granuloma will resolve satisfactorily without treatment, unless it becomes infected and requires antibiotics. Epididymitis (inflammation of the spermatic ducts between the testes and the vas) occurs in less than 1% of vasectomy cases and is treated by heat, antibiotics, and the use of an athletic supporter. Men with chronic infections such as prostatitis may be more likely to experience a postvasectomy infection.

Mortality from vasectomy is lower than that of female sterilization, estimated at 1 per 100,000 cases even under the most difficult field conditions (see Table 6-4). Tetanus and other postoperative infections are the usual cause of vasectomy-related mortality.

The only possible long-term side-effect of vasectomy that has yet been postulated is the development of spermatozoan antibodies in vasectomized men. Sperm continue to be manufactured in the testicles even after vasectomy, but without an avenue for escape, they break down. Sperm by-products are absorbed by the surrounding tissues and eventually enter the circulation. The body responds to these "foreign" substances by manufacturing *antibodies* to them, and high levels of these antibodies are found in up to two-thirds of vasectomized men. The relevance of this development is unclear.

Table 6-8. Vasectomy Complications.
• Bleeding • Infection • Hematoma • Granuloma • Epididymitis

Researchers have found significantly more atherosclerosis (deposits leading to narrowing of the arteries) in vasectomized rhesus monkeys who show high levels of antibodies than in those with low sperm antibody levels. It is assumed, but by no means proved, that there is a causal connection. Four United States studies in humans and a Danish study have failed to confirm an association between vasectomy and a subsequent increased risk of coronary disease. Nevertheless, since researchers have not been able to follow vasectomized men for long periods of time, several large-scale studies are under way to further investigate this issue.

Some physicians have suggested that in light of these preliminary monkey studies, men at high risk of cardiovascular disease should delay having a vasectomy until more research is done. This would include men with high cholesterol and triglyceride levels, diabetes, obesity, a family history of cardiovascular disease, or those who smoke. However, this position is not justified by the evidence available at the present time.

Vasectomy may produce an unexpected *benefit*, however. Preliminary research has found that women whose partners have had vasectomies have one-fourth the risk of developing cervical cancer than women whose partners are not vasectomized.

Reversibility

As with female sterilization, vasectomy should be considered *permanent* with currently available techniques. Theoretically, vasectomy can be reversed by reconnecting the cut vas (*reanastomosis*) or by using specially designed removable devices or valves to occlude the vas. None of these methods are as yet easily performed or readily available.

Surgical reanastomosis is the most effective means of reversing vasectomy presently and is actually more successful than in the female. Success—as defined by reappearance of spermatozoa in the ejaculate—has been reported in 60%–90% of cases. However, *functional* success—actually achieving pregnancy—is much harder to accomplish. Studies report functional success rates of 50%–70%. The average time from reversal of vasectomy to conception is 8 months. Apparently, the longer the man waits after the vasectomy before attempting reversal, the less likely that the reversal will be successful. There are numerous anatomical and physiological obstacles to reversal of vasectomy unrelated to the technical accomplishment of reanastomosis. Even when all the conditions are positive, reversal requires highly sophisticated surgical techniques that can be performed by specialists in a limited number of medical centers worldwide.

Various plugs, clips, threads, and valves have been tested in hopes of finding a design that could occlude the vas with minimal trauma to surrounding tissues and then could be removed or opened when the man desires restored fertility. All such designs remain experimental at this time.

For couples considering voluntary sterilization to end their childbearing, vasectomy may be the approach of choice, assuming that no contraindications exist. Vasectomy is simpler and safer than the female sterilization techniques, with equal effectiveness. However, cultural and individual acceptability may not be equal. The issues involved in choosing sterilization are discussed in the sections that follow.

CHOOSING STERILIZATION

The preceding sections of this chapter have provided the technical background with which every family planning provider should be familiar. The counselor must also be familiar with the complexity of client motivations for choosing sterilization.

Counseling

Counseling is more than the imparting of information: it is an exploration of feelings and attitudes that leads to a decision. Counseling techniques and the skills required are discussed in detail in Chapter 1. The choice for sterilization requires particular care and thoroughness in exploring risks and benefits because of the operation's permanence. In addition to the counseling session, it is particularly important that the physician actually performing the operation also speak with the patient before the procedure. The physician must be satisfied that the person undergoing sterilization fully understands the risks and its permanence.

Voluntary sterilization may be sought for many reasons, including:

- Completion of desired family size
- Desire to not have children at all
- Economic considerations
- Dislike, fear, or failure of reversible contraceptive methods
- Medical indications
- Influence of family, friends, or media

During the counseling process, the individual's reasons must be clearly identified and confirmed. One may be motivated by factors that one does not immediately recognize. The counselor and client together may find that some factors are more important than others. Even if the end result—choosing sterilization—is the same, it is psychologically important for clients to know why they are doing it. This helps to prevent postoperative misgivings or regret. Any reasons given for wanting sterilization should be deemed acceptable by the provider as long as these reasons do not demonstrate evidence of mental illness. The provider should also be wary of a client who seems confused, contradictory, or ambivalent. In these cases the counseling session must try to clarify the confusion.

Both sexual partners should be involved in the counseling process, and the decision should be a joint one if possible and appropriate. However, the provider should not *insist* on a mutual decision.

Subtle personal and family dynamics may underlie a sterilization decision, particularly when choosing which partner should be sterilized. Circumstances can change rapidly. Children may die, as may the person's sexual partner. That partner may change through death, divorce, or breakup of the relationship. The counselor must make sure that the client considers these possibilities and still chooses to no longer be able to reproduce. As another example, one partner may be significantly older than the other, or in poor health, and therefore likely to die before the other partner is no longer capable of reproduction. It may be appropriate for the older or ill partner to be sterilized (if not contraindicated) in order to allow the other to have children in a subsequent relationship.

Age and number of living children should no longer be considered absolutes in formulating criteria for approving a sterilization request. Young, unmarried, and/or childless persons will require special counseling, however, since they run a greater risk of psychological and physical dysfunction after sterilization if they later regret their decision.

The provider must strike a balance between respecting a client's motivations and trying to prevent future psychological trauma. The counselor should be alert for those who may look to sterilization as a cure for their social or personal difficulties. If ambivalence about the procedure is not resolved at the end of the counseling process, the provider should not agree to proceed with sterilization referral.

Client Education

The counselor-educator should use the information presented in the earlier sections of this chapter to prepare for explaining sterilization procedures to prospective clients. It is often helpful to give clients written materials on sterilization before the counseling session so that they can come prepared with questions.

Each person who decides on sterilization should have at least a general understanding of the operation to be performed, the possible side-effects and complications involved, and the permanence or irreversibility of the operation. The client should also be told what to expect on the day of the procedure and what postoperative care will be necessary. This is important to explain even though the actual surgical service will be providing additional instructions.

The counselor can expect to be asked questions similar to the following:

- How effective is this procedure at preventing pregnancy?
- Will I have the option to change my mind later (is it reversible)?
- What will the operation entail?
- Why has this particular procedure been recommended to me?
- How does it stop me from having babies (or making someone pregnant)?
- Will I be hospitalized?
- Will it hurt?
- What kind of scar will it leave?
- What are the physical risks and how likely are they to occur?
- If I do get pregnant later despite this, will it be dangerous?

Most of these questions have been answered above. Although sterilization is very effective, the client should understand that it is not *guaranteed* effective. The risks of sterilization should be fully explained and yet put into some kind of perspective that the client can readily understand, such as the risks of other operations, other contraceptive methods, or childbearing.

The counselor should also expect questions of a more personal nature. To most people, even those most strongly motivated, the concept of sterilization can seem to threaten their sexuality. Both men and women need to be sensitively reassured about their continuing capacity for sexual fulfillment after sterilization. The man still ejaculates semen after vasectomy and will not find his ability to have an erection affected. The woman, too, should understand that only her tubes have been affected and not her hormones or sexual feelings. Some women also may not realize that their menstrual periods will continue, and they can be reassured that menopause will not occur earlier. Both men and women will be pleased to hear that the scars left by laparoscopy, minilaparotomy, and vasectomy are small. The resolution of these psychological issues may have much more to do with the client choosing sterilization than the client learning about details of operative technique.

Timing

Sterilization procedures can be performed at essentially any time. "Interval" sterilization—not associated with a recent delivery or abortion—is increasingly popular. Female sterilization can be performed immediately postpartum or postabortion, but these are not always periods when the woman can make a relaxed and informed choice. If a woman has an unwanted pregnancy and wishes to be sterilized, an abortion will have to be performed first, of course, but they can be done concurrently.

Women choosing sterilization who are using barrier methods or IUDs should continue these methods right up to the time of the operation in order to avoid a last-minute pregnancy. Oral contraceptive users should complete the cycle of pills they are taking, even if this means taking pills after the sterilization procedure, in order to maintain hormonal regularity.

A couple may decide to end childbearing after learning that the woman is pregnant, and in doing so may be counting on a normal delivery. In these instances it is best to postpone the decision for vasectomy or postpartum sterilization until after the health of the newborn is assured.

Choice of Procedure

The initial choice for a couple considering sterilization is which partner will be sterilized. Vasectomy is simpler, safer, and just as effective as female sterilization. Consequently, it is the method of choice, all other factors being equal.

The choice of a female sterilization approach will probably be made by the surgeon after the referral. The selection will be determined by the presence of any contraindications, the timing (postpartum, for instance), and the availability of equipment and personnel. The final choice of approach and the reasons for it should be explained to the woman.

Referral

When the counselor is satisfied that the client has made a fully informed choice for sterilization, the counselor should arrange to refer the client to a sterilization provider. Often, but not always, this will mean sending the client to another facility. As with all referral procedures, the counselor should be confident of the surgeon's skill, safety, and sensitivity. The client's medical and contraceptive history should be forwarded to the surgical facility, along with documentation of the counseling session and its conclusion. Depending on the procedures used, an *informed consent* form will be signed with either the counseling service, the surgical service, or both (see below).

The family planning provider who does not offer sterilization personally should not consider the moment of referral as the end of involvement with the client. Whenever possible, the provider should stay in contact with the client through the sterilization procedure and offer to assist the client in any way necessary up to and after the procedure.

Informed Consent

In medical practice, the concept of "informed consent" has come to mean the written documentation that a patient has been fully informed about the nature of a procedure and its intended effects and possible side-effects and complications. Informed consent is particularly critical for a sterilization procedure because of its far-reaching consequences. Thus at the appropriate point in the preoperative process, the patient must sign a consent form that documents that his or her choice of sterilization is informed and voluntary.

Every service offering sterilization must develop administrative procedures to ensure that no client is ever coerced or induced to choose sterilization. Guidelines are necessary to protect the rights of public assistance recipients, minors, or the mentally incompetent. The rights of health providers should also be protected, so that no one is required to perform or assist with sterilization procedures if this is contrary to their personal convictions.

Postoperative Reactions

Despite the best efforts at preoperative counseling and the most sincere and enthusiastic client motivations, a small number of sterilization patients will experience adverse psychological effects after the procedure. These effects can range from a very limited short-term depression or feeling of regret immediately after the operation to serious mental disturbances. Those reactions at the more mild end of the scale are relatively common, but serious side-effects are rare and can often by prevented by proper client screening and a clear exploration of feelings before the operation.

It has been estimated that less than 5% of all persons who choose sterilization will later regret their decision. The probability of regret is certainly higher when the decision is made in the midst of an unhappy marriage or similar strong emotional upset. Regret also seems to be more common when the decision is made immediately after a pregnancy, or when the woman is under 30 years old. On the other hand, the frequency of regret seems to be lower among young nulliparous women who are committed to having no children at all. Thus family planning providers should not assume that a request for sterilization from such a women will mean a high risk of postoperative problems. In general, most researchers agree that there are too many unpredictable circumstances in anyone's life—death, divorce, and so on—to meaningfully predict postoperative regret.

Because these rare psychological reactions are so unfortunate, it must be emphasized again that providers counseling clients for sterilization should be cautious in allowing sterilization to be chosen by clients who are strongly ambivalent or exhibit significant emotional disturbance.

Selected Readings

Alder E, Cook A, Gray J, et al: The effects of sterilization: A comparison of sterilized women with the wives of vasectomised men. Contraception 23(1): 45, January 1981

Alexander I: The timing of laparoscopic sterilization in relation to prior contraception. The British Journal of Family Planning 6(3): 69, October 1980

Alexander NJ: Evaluating the safety of vasectomy. Fertility and Sterility 37(6): 734, June 1982

Alexander NJ, Clarkson TB: Vasectomy increases the severity of diet-induced atherosclerosis in *Macaca fascicularis*. Science 201: 538, 1978

Alexander NJ, Clarkson TB: Long-term vasectomy: Effects on the occurrence and extent of atherosclerosis in rhesus monkeys. Journal of Clinical Investigation 65: 15, 1980

Anonymous: New finding added to debate on postvasectomy semen examination regimen. Network 1(3): 2, May 1980

Anonymous: Vasectomy reversal. Lancet 2: 625, September 20, 1980

Anonymous: Contraceptive Technology Update 1(6): 77, September 1980 (sterilization issue)

Anonymous: Mortality risks associated with female procedures: A summary of the IPAVS experience. IPAVS Newsletter No. 25, February 1981

Anonymous: Reversal of female sterilization. AVS Biomedical Bulletin 2(2): 1, July 1981

Anonymous: Vasectomy reversal success variable. Contraceptive Technology Update, March 1982

Aranda C, Broutin A, Edelman D, et al: A comparative study of electrocoagulation and tubal rings for tubal occlusion at laparoscopy. International Journal of Gynecology and Obstetrics 14(5): 411, 1976

Aubert JM, Lubell I, Schima M: Mortality risk associated with female sterilization. International Journal of Gynecology and Obstetrics 18(6): 406, 1980

Baggish MS, Lee WK, Miro SJ, et al: Complications of laparoscopic sterilization. Obstetrics and Gynecology 54(1): 54, July 1979

Bedford JM, Zelikovsky G: Viability of spermatoza in the human ejaculate after vasectomy. Fertility and Sterility 32(4): 460, October 1979

Bhatt RV, Pachauri S, Pathak ND, et al: A comparative study of the tubal ring applied via minilaparotomy and laparoscopy in postabortion cases. International Journal of Gynecology and Obstetrics 16(2): 162, 1978

Bhiwandiwala PP, Mumford SD, Feldblum PJ: Menstrual pattern changes following laparoscopic sterilization. Obstetrics and Gynecology 27(5): 249, May 1982

Bhiwandiwala PP, Mumford SD, Feldblum PJ: A comparison of different laparoscopic sterilization occlusion techniques in 24,439 procedures. American Journal of Obstetrics and Gynecology 144(3): 319, October 1, 1982

Bradshaw LE: Vasectomy reversibility—a status report. Population Reports D(3): 41, Washington DC, George Washington University, May 1976

Burkman RT, Magarick RH, Waife RS (eds): Surgical Equipment and Training in Reproductive Health. Baltimore, JHPIEGO, 1980, 120 pp

Chi I, Feldblum P: Uterine perforation during steriization by laparoscopy and minilaparotomy. American Journal of Obstetrics and Gynecology 139(4): 735, March 15, 1981

Chi I, Feldblum P: Laparoscopic sterilizations requiring laparotomy. American Journal of Obstetrics and Gynecology 142(6): 712, March 15, 1982

Chi I, Laufe LE, Gardner SD, et al: An epidemiologic study of risk factors associated with pregnancy following female sterilization. American Journal of Obstetrics and Gynecology 136(6): 768, March 15, 1980

Cooper P, et al: Psychological sequelae to elective sterilization: A prospective study. British Medical Journal 284: 461, February 13, 1982

Cunanan RG, Courey NG, Lippes J: Complications of laparoscopic tubal sterilization. Obstetrics and Gynecology 55(4): 501, April 1980

Davis J, de Castro MP, Mumford SD: Consensus on vasectomy. Lancet 2: 1222, November 27, 1982

Decherney AH, Mezer H, Naftolin F: Failure of surgical reanastomosis following tubal ligation. Fertility and Sterility 37(2): 291, February 1982

DeStefano F, Peterson HB, Layde PM, et al: Risk of ectopic pregnancy following tubal sterilization. Obstetrics and Gynecology 60(3): 326, September 1982

Domenzain ME, Gonsalez MA, Teran J: Minilaparotomy tubal sterilization: A comparison between normal and high-risk patients. Obstetrics and Gynecology 59(2): 199, February 1982

Dusitsin N, Boonsiri B, Chitpatima K: Bangkok: Are males resistant to sterilization? International Family Planning Perspectives 6(1): 26, March 1980

Gomel V: Profile of women requesting reversal of sterilization. Fertility and Sterility 30(1): 39, July 1978

Gomel V: Microsurgical reversal of female sterilization: A reappraisal. Fertility and Sterility 33(6): 587, June 1980

Green CP: Voluntary sterilization: World's leading contraceptive method. Population Reports, Baltimore, Population Information Program, March 1978

Henry A, Rinehart W, Piotrow PT: Reversing female sterilization. Population Reports C(8), Baltimore, Population Information Program, September 1980

Johnson JH: Tubal sterilization and hysterectomy. Family Planning Perspectives 14(1): 28, January/February 1982

Kessel E, Mumford SD: Potential demand for voluntary female sterilization in the 1980s: The compelling need for a nonsurgical method. Fertility and Sterility 37(6): 725, June 1982

Koetsawang S, Srisupandit S, Cole LP: Laparoscopic electrocoagulation and tubal ring techniques for sterilization: A comparative study. International Journal of Gynecology and Obstetrics 15(5): 455, 1978

Lee RB, Boyd JAK: Minilaparotomy under local anesthesia for outpatient sterilization: A preliminary report. Fertility and Sterility 33(2): 129, February 1980

Limpaphayom K, Reinprayoon D, Aribarg A, et al: Laparoscopic tubal electrocoagulation for sterilization: 5000 cases. International Journal of Gynecology and Obstetrics 18(6): 411, 1980

Linnet L, Moller NPH, Bernth-Petersen P, et al: No increase in arteriosclerotic retinopathy or activity in tests for circulating immune complexes 5 years after vasectomy. Fertility and Sterility 37(6): 798, June 1982

Loffer FD, Pent D: Pregnancy after laparoscopic sterilization. Obstetrics and Gynecology 55(5): 643, May 1980

Lynn SC, Katz AR, Ross PJ: Aortic perforation sustained at laparoscopy. Journal of Reproductive Medicine 27(4): 217, April 1982

McCann MF, Kessel E: International experience with laparoscopic sterilization: Follow-up of 8500 women. Advances in Planned Parenthood 12(4): 199, 1978

Mumford SD, Bhiwandiwala PP, Chi I: Laparscopic and minilaparotomy female sterilization compared in 15,167 cases. Lancet 2: 1066, November 15, 1980

Penfield AJ: Open laparoscopy, in Burkman RT, Magarick RH, Waife RS (eds): Surgical Equipment and Training in Reproductive Health. Baltimore, JHPIEGO, 1980, p 17

Peterson HB, DeStefano F, Greenspan JR, et al: Mortality risk associated with tubal sterilization in United States hospitals. American Journal of Obstetrics and Gynecology 143(2): 125, May 15, 1982

Peterson HB, Greenspan JR, DeStefano F, et al: Deaths associated with laparoscopic sterilization in the United States, 1977–79. Journal of Reproductive Medicine 27(6): 345, June 1982

Peterson HB, Greenspan JR, Ory HW: Death following puncture of the aorta during laparosopic sterilization. Obstetrics and Gynecology 59(1): 133, January 1982

Peterson HB, Ory HW, Greenspan JR, et al: Deaths associated with laparoscopic sterilization by unipolar electrocoagulating devices, 1978 and 1979. American Journal of Obstetrics and Gynecology 139(2): 141, January 15, 1981

Porter CW, Hulka JF: Female sterilization in current practice. Family Planning Perspectives 6(1): 30, Winter 1974

Quigley HJ, Lacy S, Curtis G: Atherosclerosis in vasectomized rabbits. Fertility and Sterility 37(2): 321, February 1982

Radwanska E, Headley SK, Dmowski P: Evaluation of ovarian function after tubal sterilization. Journal of Reproductive Medicine 27(7): 376, July 1982

Schima ME, Lubell I: Voluntary Sterilization: A Decade of Achievement. New York, Association for Voluntary Sterilization, 1980

Swan SH, Brown WL: Vasectomy and cancer of the cervix. The New England Journal of Medicine 301(1): 46, July 5, 1979

Tatum HJ, Schmidt FH: Contraceptive and sterilization practices and extrauterine pregnancy: A realistic perspective. Fertility and Sterility 28(4): 407, April 1977

Walker AM, Hunter JR, Watkins RN, et al: Vasectomy and non-fatal myocardial infarction. Lancet 1: 13, January 3, 1981

Walker AM, Jick H, Hunter JR, et al: Hospitalization rates in vasectomized men. Journal of the American Medical Association 245(22): 2315, June 12, 1981

Wallace RB, Lee J, Gerber WL, et al: Vasectomy and coronary disease in men under 50: Absence of an association. Journal of Urology 126(8): 182, 1981

World Health Organization: Sequelae of vasectomy. Contraception 25(2): 119, February 1982

World Health Organization: Minilaparotomy of laparoscopy for sterilization: A multicenter, multinational randomized study. American Journal of Obstetrics and Gynecology 143(6): 645, July 15, 1982

Wortman J: Female sterilization by minilaparotomy. Population Reports C(5), Washington, DC, George Washington University, November 1974

Wortman J, Piotrow PT: Vasectomy: Old and new techniques. Population Report D(1), Washington, DC, George Washington University, December 1973

Referral for Other Health Problems

7

Health practitioners providing contraceptive care may frequently find that their clients have other health problems. Family planning is a part of health care; it would be difficult—and unprofessional— to ignore these other physical disorders. Moreover, family planning clients will appreciate the provider's concern for their other health problems.

Sometimes, family planning providers properly trained in health care can treat the conditions discussed in this chapter themselves. But the context of this chapter is *referral*: it is assumed that some other provider, usually a specialized physician, will be needed. When the nonphysician family planning provider can start treatment, it is so indicated. All these conditions will require more or less prompt attention. Gynecological, sexually transmitted, and other common health problems are listed.

Every family planning facility should have a list of appropriate referral sources and guidelines for referring clients. A cooperative arrangement should be established so that the referral source will be expecting new patients. It is desirable for the referring provider to help the client with any procedural details and even assist in transportation if necessary. As with all referrals, the family planning provider should carefully check the quality of the referral resource and regularly monitor the appropriateness of its care.

The most critical referral resource needed is a facility for emergency care. Even a clinic exclusively devoted to family planning will occasionally see critically ill patients. In this context, the family planning provider should remember that the community is likely to consider *any* health service as comprehensive and, therefore, should acknowledge the professional responsibility to handle these emergencies through referral.

Whenever a person presents with an undiagnosed health problem, one of the first questions a practitioner should ask is what method of contraception the person is using, if any. This is particularly important in women with gynecological, abdominal, or circulatory symptoms. The family planning provider can serve as an important source of information in these referral situations, since that person is more likely than the referral physician to know about the relevance of the contraceptive method to the health problem.

GYNECOLOGICAL CONDITIONS

During the course of history-taking or physical examination for the provision of contraception, one will frequently encounter gynecological problems. The first two listed here—pelvic inflammatory disease (PID) and ectopic pregnancy—will require immediate attention, and have been discussed often in previous chapters.

Pelvic Inflammatory Disease

Women may be seen with multiple complaints of lower abdominal pain, fever, vaginal discharge, and/or painful intercourse. Usually these symptoms of pelvic inflammation occur following a menstrual period. On examination there is often a foul-smelling vaginal discharge and extreme uterine tenderness when the cervix is moved. The adnexae are often tender and a tuboovarian mass may be present. Pelvic inflammatory disease is more likely to be seen in women using an IUD and is less likely to be seen in oral contraceptive users. If the patient is using an IUD, it should be removed without delay.

The family planning provider can consider treating uncomplicated PID without referral by starting the woman on appropriate antibiotics. She should be seen again within 24–48 hours, and if there is no improvement, she should be referred for more extensive diagnosis and treatment. But if the provider is uncertain about providing any treatment, referral should be made immediately. Pelvic inflammatory disease is discussed in detail in Chapter 3.

Ectopic Pregnancy

A woman with an ectopic (tubal) pregnancy will often complain first of an abnormal menstrual period, followed by persistent vaginal bleeding and the onset of abdominal pain or tenderness. In contrast to PID, women with an ectopic pregnancy seldom have a fever, and pain is usually more pronounced on one side of the abdomen. On examination there may be a palpable tender adnexal mass on one side. Ectopic pregnancy should also be suspected when a pregnancy test is positive but physical examination does not reveal an intrauterine pregnancy.

In ectopic pregnancy there is the potential of the affected fallopian tube bursting, causing life-threating intraabdominal bleeding. The danger can be quite sudden, and thus any suspicion of ectopic pregnancy requires immediate referral. The relationship of ectopic pregnancy to IUD use and pregnancy termination is discussed in Chapters 3 and 5.

Breast Masses

Most women of reproductive age are concerned about the possibility of developing breast masses. Breast palpation is often performed by a family planning provider as part of the general physical examination. Whereas most breast masses are benign, any woman who is found to have a lump in her breast may have cancer and should be referred to a physician for evaluation. The three most common types of breast masses are fibrocystic disease, fibroadenomas, and breast cancer.

Fibrocystic disease. In this benign condition the breast often has multiple lumps and a nodular feeling. This is most pronounced just before menstruation and may be associated with discomfort and a sense of fullness in the breast. If the women is reexamined after menstruation, the nodularity will usually be significantly diminished. Aspiration of fluid from cysts in the breast may be used to confirm the diagnosis of fibrocystic disease. The condition is most common among women 30–40 years old. Although fibrocystic disease is a benign condition, it is associated with a slightly increased risk of breast cancer. The use of oral contraceptives apparently lowers the risk of developing benign breast disease. Preexisting fibrocystic disease is not a contraindication to pill use.

Table 7-1.
Risk Factors for Breast Cancer.
• 40–60 years of age • Strong family history of breast cancer   (mother, sister, maternal aunt)

Fibroadenoma. Fibroadenomas are another type of benign breast mass. In general they are smooth, firm, painless masses that are movable and distinct from the surrounding breast tissue. There may be multiple masses in one breast. Fibroadenomas may be seen in women under 30.

Breast cancer. Women with breast cancer usually have a firm painless mass that is fixed to the adjacent breast tissue. In more advanced cancer, there may be redness, swelling, or retraction of the skin overlying the mass, and axillary lymph nodes (under the arm) may be palpable. The most common location for breast cancer is in the lateral quadrants (the left side of the left breast, and the right side of the right breast), but lesions can occur anywhere in the breasts. The age group for peak occurrence of breast cancer is 40–60 years old; women with a strong family history of breast cancer (in the mother, sister, or maternal aunt) are at especially high risk (Table 7-1). Oral contraceptive users do not have an increased risk of breast cancer. Preexisting breast cancer is an absolute contraindication to pill use because the growth and spread of the cancer can be increased by hormonal stimulation.

Uterine Fibroids

Uterine fibroids will often be detected during a routine pelvic examination—approximately one-fourth of all women have them to some degree. Fibroids are benign "fibromuscular" growths that arise within the uterine musculature, causing irregular distortion and enlargement of the uterus (Figure 7-1). Fibroids are usually found in women in their thirties but may also occur in younger women. Although they are occasionally asymptomatic, fibroids are often associated with lower abdominal discomfort and pressure, heavy menstrual bleeding, and cramps. Almost all uterine fibroids are benign; less than 1% are malignant.

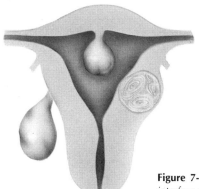

Figure 7-1. *Uterine fibroids are usually benign but may interfere with the effectiveness of an IUD.*

Fibroids should be suspected if the uterus of a nonpregnant women is enlarged and irregular. Barrier contraceptives are the most appropriate family planning method for women with fibroids. The effectiveness of an IUD will be reduced in the presence of fibroids because of the distortion of the uterine cavity.

Endometriosis

Endometriosis occurs when "islands" of endometrial tissue, similar to the lining of the uterus, are found implanted outside of the uterus, in the pelvic cavity. Endometriosis most commonly occurs in women 25–40 years old, particularly those who have not had children. Endometriosis may be asymptomatic but is usually associated with pain prior to and during menstruation, painful intercourse, and/or rectal pain and diarrhea during menstruation.

Endometriosis can worsen and cause infertility. Consequently, contraceptive clients with this condition who desire to have children in the future may want to consider childbearing earlier than planned. Oral contraceptives may reduce the symptoms of endometriosis but should be used for this purpose only under the close supervision of a physician.

Ovarian Cysts

Ovarian cysts are also found on routine pelvic examination (Figure 7-2). Cysts may be asymptomatic but are often associated with irregular menstrual bleeding, abdominal pain, a sense of abdominal fullness, and uncomfortable intercourse. They may be benign or ma-

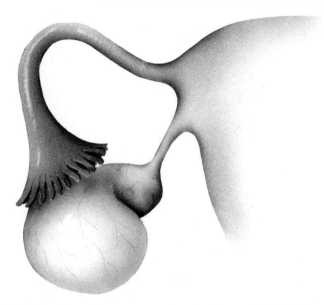

Figure 7-2. *Oral contraceptives are apparently protective against the development of ovarian cysts.*

lignant; in general, the risk of malignancy increases with age. The most common ovarian cysts occurring in younger women are benign cysts that increase in size before the menstrual period and usually recede afterward. If the woman is under age 30 and the cyst is estimated to be 5 cm or less in diameter, it is probably sufficient to follow her for several cycles to see whether the cyst disappears. If the cyst persists, is over 5 cm, or if the woman is over 40, the patient should be referred to a physician promptly.

Oral contraceptive use appears to be protective against the development of benign ovarian cysts. Consequently, if a cyst is found in a pill user, the odds that it is caused by a disease are greater, demanding immediate physician referral. Pill use does not in any way *cause* the development of ovarian disease and appears to be protective against the development of ovarian cancer.

Cervical Abnormalities

A wide variety of cervical abnormalities may be noted on pelvic examination. *Nabothian cysts* (benign cysts under the cervical surface) are extremely common and may distort the cervix. No treatment is necessary. *Cervicitis* (cervical infection) may be identified by cervical irritation and profuse foul discharge. A culture should be taken to rule out the presence of gonorrhea (see page 274). If that culture is negative, the treatment for cervicitis is sulfa vaginal creams or oral antibiotics. Cryocautery (freezing of the cervix) may also be beneficial.

Cervical dysplasias or malignancy may be discovered at the family planning clinic. Routine screening for these conditions by Papanicolaou (Pap) smears should be performed when possible. If any abnormalities are found on Pap smear, the woman should be referred for gynecological evaluation. Evaluation may be made by colposcopy (cervical examination with a magnifying instrument) or biopsy (removing a portion of tissue for microscopic examination). No contraceptive methods cause cervical dysplasia or malignancy. Oral contraceptives may promote the progression of *preexisting* dysplasia to carcinoma in situ. Patients with cervical dysplasia should be followed closely by repeat Pap smears.

Bartholin's Cysts

Bartholin's glands are mucus-secreting glands in the labia minora that may become plugged, leading to development of a cyst or an abscess. A Bartholin's cyst is usually an enlarged, soft mass within one of the labia minora. If the cyst becomes infected, an abscess can form, leading to redness, swelling, and tenderness. Cysts do not require treatment if they remain asymptomatic. Abscesses are usually treated with hot soaks and antibiotics. Incision and drainage may be necessary if the abscess is large and well established or if it does not respond to antibiotics.

Toxic Shock Syndrome

Toxic shock syndrome is a bacterial infection caused by *Staphylococcus aureus*. This syndrome is most frequently seen in women under 25 years of age during menstruation, but it has also been identified among nonmenstruating women, men, and children in some cases.

Definitive diagnosis of toxic shock syndrome can be difficult, but six symptoms present most frequently: fever of 102°F (39°C) or greater, hypotension or dizziness, rash or desquamation (shedding of skin) a week to 10 days after onset of the disease, and involvement of at least three other body systems, including the gastrointestinal, muscular, mucous membrane, renal, hepatic, or central nervous systems. When a preponderance of these symptoms are manifest in a patient, particularly a menstruating woman, the patient should be referred for differential diagnosis and treatment. Prompt treatment of toxic shock syndrome with antibiotics is important because recurrence of the syndrome in untreated cases can be more severe than the initial episode.

Toxic shock syndrome has been associated with the use of high-absorbency tampons, regardless of name brand. Lower-absorbency tampons also slightly increase the incidence of toxic shock syndrome but not nearly as significantly. Women with symptoms of toxic shock syndrome should discontinue any tampon use until after diagnosis and treatment. Research indicates no relationship beween toxic shock syndrome and any of the following: duration of tampon use, number of tampons used per day, contraceptive method used (including diaphragms and cervical caps), sexual history, or history of sexually transmitted diseases.

VAGINAL AND URINARY INFECTIONS

Because vaginal and urinary infections can be considered both gynecological and sexually associated, they are discussed together in this section, before focusing on sexually transmitted diseases. Vaginal and urinary infections plague all women frequently, and occasionally men will have a urethral infection. These conditions will be seen regularly by the family planning provider. Most of these conditions can be treated without referral, although access to laboratory facilities is usually required.

Vaginal Infections

Vaginal infections are categorized by the causative organisms: nonspecific vaginitis, trichomonas vaginitis, and yeast (candida) vaginitis (Table 7-2).

Nonspecific vaginitis. Nonspecific vaginitis is caused by a variety of organisms, including *Hemophilus vaginalis*, *Chlamydia trachomatis* (see page 270), and others. It may also be caused by frequent douching, chemical irritation from the use of feminine hygiene products, or emotional stress. The discharge is variably gray-green to yellow in color and may be thick or watery. Vaginal itching and burning may be present but usually are not pronounced; there may be pain on urination. A fishy odor is often associated with a discharge of this type. Diagnosis can be made by a microscopic examination of a wet mount saline preparation of the vaginal secretions. If no trichomonas or yeast are seen, the infection is presumed to be "nonspecific." When the causative organism is *Hemophilus vaginalis*, numerous bacteria and "clue cells" (stippled vaginal epithelial cells overlain with bacteria) may be seen. A culture or Gram stain for gonorrhea can be performed to rule the possibility of gonococcal infection.

The most common treatment for nonspecific vaginal discharge is sulfa-containing vaginal creams or suppositories. In some instances, the use of oral metronidazole (Flagyl) or tetracycline may be beneficial.

Trichomonas vaginitis. Trichomonas vaginitis is a sexually transmitted infection caused by *Trichomonas vaginalis*. Symptoms may occur 4–28 days after exposure. Women with trichomonas infection usually complain of vaginal discharge and itching; burning on urination is also sometimes present. Examination will reveal a profuse frothy greenish vaginal discharge. On close inspection, small red areas on the vagina and cervix ("strawberry red spots") may sometimes be seen. Trichomonas may be readily diagnosed by microscopic examination of a wet mount saline preparation of the vaginal discharge. The *Trichomonas vaginalis* organisms are slightly larger than white blood cells and have a jerking motion caused by their rapidly moving flagella (Figure 7-3). The treatment is metronidazole (Flagyl). Whenever possible, both sexual partners should be treated at the same time so that trichomonas will not be reintroduced from one partner to the other.

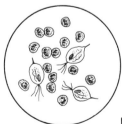

Figure 7-3. *Trichomonas.*

Table 7-2. Vaginal Infections.		
Type of Infection	Incubation	Symptoms
Nonspecific vaginitis	Indefinite	Discharge and pain, sometimes on urination
Hemophilus	Indefinite	Discharge; odor and irritation
Trichomonas	4–28 days	Greenish yellow discharge; pain and burning
Candida (yeast)	Indefinite	White, clumpy discharge; pain and burning

Yeast (candida) vaginitis. Yeast (candida) vaginitis exhibits a discharge with a lumpy white "cottage cheese" appearance and is often associated with redness of the labia and intense itching. The presence of yeast may be diagnosed microscopically by a wet-mount saline preparation or a special potassium hydroxide preparation of the vaginal secretions. The yeast also can be cultured in a special medium. The treatment for yeast infections is nystatin (Mycostatin) suppositories or other vaginal preparations such as miconazole cream (Monistat) or clotrimazole cream or suppositories (Gyne-Lotrimin). If infection is persistent, treatment with oral nystatin may be useful for elimination of a possible reservoir of yeast in the gastrointestinal tract. Topical acidifying creams or gentian violet for the vagina are also sometimes used.

Yeast infections may result from antibiotic use, pregnancy, or diabetes. Any women with frequent occurrences of unexplained yeast infections should be evaluated for possible glucose intolerance. Finally, those women with yeast infections who are using a high-potency progestin pill formulation such as Ovral may benefit from a change to another oral contraceptive with relatively less progestin dominance (see page 43).

Diagnostic Procedure	Treatment	Complications
Difficult; rule out gonorrhea by culture	Tetracycline; erythromycin	Reinfection from untreated partner
Culture: identification of "clue cells"	Metronidazole	Reinfection from untreated partner
Slide and culture	Metronidazole	Reinfection from untreated partner
Slide and culture	Clotrimazole; miconazole	Reinfection from untreated partner

Urinary Tract Infections

Urinary tract infections (UTI) can involve the kidneys or bladder, but often affect only the urethra. In women the most common form of UTI involves both the bladder and the urethra (*cystitis*); in men the most common UTI affects only the urethra (see below). Urinary tract infections occur more frequently in women than in men as a result of anatomical differences: women have a shorter urethra whose opening is close to the vaginal and anal orifices.

Urine provides an ideal medium for bacterial growth. Symptoms of UTI typically include some combination of the following: burning on urination, frequent urination in small amounts, "urgency" (the need to urinate immediately), lower abdominal or middle back pain, blood in the urine, and/or unusually dark, cloudy, or foul-smelling urine. These symptoms may be accompanied by systemic signs of infection such as fever and chills.

Whenever possible, a urinalysis should be conducted to determine the specific causative bacteria in order to choose the appropriate antibiotic. After therapy, a second urinalysis should be conducted to confirm elimination of the bacteria.

Nongonococcal urethritis. Nongonococcal urethritis (NGU), also referred to as nonspecific urethritis (NSU), is a urinary tract infection in males that is usually sexually associated. Nongonococcal urethritis is a urethral inflammation characterized by burning and/or itching upon urination and a thin, almost clear discharge or "drip." Diagnosis of urethritis in the male is more complicated than in the female because the symptoms closely resemble those of gonorrhea. Whereas only a laboratory culture can positively rule out gonorrhea, most frequently NGU is caused by chlamydia. Unfortunately, chlamydia is difficult to culture (only 14 centers in the United States can do so, for instance), and as a result chlamydia usually remains unidentified.

Public health officials have confirmed that there is an epidemic of chlamydial infections in the United States and Sweden, and they are likely to be prevalent elsewhere. Sexual transmission to the female can be dangerous; if undiagnosed or untreated, chlamydial infection can lead to pelvic inflammatory disease (PID) and infertility, cause stillbirth in pregnant women and affect the newborn if it is delivered through an infected vagina. Consequently, although NGU is certainly a less serious condition than gonorrhea, especially for the male, it must be treated promptly.

Tetracycline or erythromycin seem to be the best antibiotic choices for nonspecific urethritis; metronidazole (Flagyl) can be used subsequently if symptoms continue and a trichomonas infection is suspected. Since chlamydial infections in women are usually asymptomatic, it is recommended that the man's sexual partner(s) be treated simultaneously to prevent possible reinfection.

SEXUALLY TRANSMITTED DISEASES

The following conditions are sexually transmitted diseases (STD) that are usually found in both men and women (see also Table 7-3). Several of them are reaching epidemic proportions, especialy genital herpes and gonorrhea. Family planning providers will often be the first and sometimes the only health providers to see people with these diseases and therefore can play a critically important role in the improvement of public health by treating or referring these clients promptly. All family planning providers should be thoroughly familiar with STD symptoms.

Genital Herpes

Herpes infections of the genitialia are increasingly referred to as an epidemic in the United States. They will be frequently seen in the family planning clinic and are caused by herpes simplex viruses (usually Type II, but occasionally Type I) transmitted through sexual contact. Approximately 3–20 days after exposure, women may develop multiple painful blisters on the labia, which break down and form ulcerated areas after several days. Whereas men can develop herpes on the penis or in the urethra, the process is usually less extensive and hence less painful than the infections in women. The sores usually heal spontaneously within 1–4 weeks, but after an initial attack of herpes, the virus remains in the nerve roots supplying the affected area. Recurrent episodes of symptomatic infection may occur, especially when the patient is ill or under stress. The diagnosis of herpes can sometimes be confirmed by taking a scraping for Pap smear from an active sore. More frequently, herpes are diagnosed visually by the clinician.

The treatment of herpes is symptomatic, as there is no known cure. Women with active herpes infections may apply cold compresses with Domeboro solution (modified Burow's solution). Pain medication is given for discomfort, and antibiotics may be useful in preventing secondary infection. A topical treatment containing acyclovir (Zovirax) is now available that can somewhat alleviate the symptoms of an initial infection but does not prevent the recurrence of herpes or alleviate the effects of a recurrence.

Any patient with active herpes lesions is extremely contagious and should refrain from intercourse for several weeks after complete healing has occurred. During this period, condoms can be used to inhibit transmission. Cervical carcinoma has been associated with a history of herpes Type II infections, and thus it is especially advisable for women with herpes to have regular annual Pap smears.

Venereal Warts

Venereal warts (condylomata) are caused by a papilloma virus and are sexually transmitted. They develop 1–3 months after exposure and, when small, are relatively painless warts with a roughened surface. Warts are dry when located externally but are moist on internal surfaces such as the urethra, vagina, or cervix. Condylomata may grow and coalesce to form a cauliflowerlike appearance, associated with irritation. In males, warts may occur on the penis and scrotum, around the anus, or in the urethra. If they block the

Table 7-3.
Sexually Transmitted Diseases.

Disease	Incubation	Symptoms
Genital herpes	3–20 days	Painful blisters around genitals that break
Venereal warts	1–3 months or longer	Irritation locally; sometimes pain
Crab lice	24–72 hours	Itching, often intense, particularly in pubic hair, chest hair, or axillary hair
Gonorrhea	3–10 days	85% of women have no symptoms; 40% of men have no symptoms; if any, discharge, burning on urination
Syphilis	40–90 days	*Painless* ulcers will go away on their own; later, rash, balding, fever, lesions, may occur
Lymphogranuloma venereum (LCV)	1–3 weeks	Painful vesicles at site of infections; swollen lymph nodes; chronic abscesses
Chancroid	1 week	Painful lesion that exudes pus; swollen lymph nodes in groin

Diagnostic Technique	Treatment	Complications
Visual and culture	Symptomatic pain relief: Acyclovir, Burrow's solution	Increased incidence of cervical cancer in women
Cauliflowerlike appearance; dry with rough surface	Podophyllin applications; occasionally cryocautery	Possible urethral blockage
Reddish dust and clear yellowish lice	Topical lindane (γ-benzene hexachloride)	None
Gram stain and culture	Penicillin G; tetracycline hcl; amoxicillin with probenecid	Can cause sterility if untreated
VDRL; dark-field microscopy	Penicillin G; erythromycin	Can cause sterility and/or severe heart and nervous system damage if untreated
Frei skin test or LGV blood test	Tetracycline or sulfa drugs	Increased incidence of rectal cancer
Gram stain; dark-field microscopy	Oral sulfa drugs; tetracycline; erythromycin	

urethra, they may require surgical removal. In females, venereal warts may be located on the vulva, vagina, and cervix and in the perianal area. On occasion, venereal warts may be confused with condylomata lata of secondary syphilis. If there is any question, a blood test (serology) should be obtained to rule out the presence of syphilis (see page 275).

The treatment for venereal warts is podophyllum, a solution that is applied to the warts once or twice weekly. This can be done at the family planning clinic. If the warts do not respond after several treatments, the patient should be referred to a physician for consideration of alternative therapy, including electrocoagulation and cryocautery (freezing).

Crab Lice

Crab lice infestations (*Phthirus pubis*) may be seen by the family planning provider. Infection with crab lice is usually transmitted sexually but may also result from sharing a bed, clothing, or towels with an infected person. Symptoms generally occur within 24–48 hours after transmission. The infestation causes intense itching in the pubic hair area. It is diagnosed visually with a magnifying glass by finding the lice or egg cases ("nits") at the base of hair shafts (Figure 7-4). The treatment of choice is gamma benzene hexachloride (Kwell) lotion, cream, or shampoo. A pyrethin solution (RID, A-200) can also be effective.

Gonorrhea

Gonorrhea is likely to be diagnosed in men and women at the family planning clinic. Approximately 85% of women with gonorrhea will be asymptomatic. When symptoms do occur, they include a purulent discharge with associated pelvic pain and fever, usually fol-

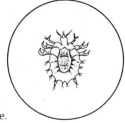

Figure 7-4. *Crab louse.*

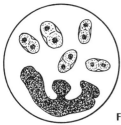

Figure 7-5. *Gonorrhea is epidemic in many countries.*

lowing menstruation. Men with gonorrhea often develop a creamy urethral discharge, usually 3–5 days after exposure, with associated pain and burning on urination. As many as 40% of males with gonorrhea are also asymptomatic, however. Gonorrhea is a serious disease, which if untreated can lead to sterility in both females and males. If gonorrhea is suspected, a culture should be taken when laboratory facilities are available. Alternately, a microscopic smear can be performed to confirm the presence of Gram-negative intracellular diplococci (Figure 7-5).

If gonorrhea is confirmed, physician referral is required. Treatment with penicillin or tetracycline will be indicated. In recent years, several strains of penicillin-resistant gonorrhea have been identified. Frequently penicillin-resistant strains of gonorrhea will respond to spectinomycin. A critical aspect of gonorrhea control is the identification and treatment of sexual partners to prevent reinfection and further spreading of the disease.

Syphilis

Syphilis is caused by a spirochete, *Treponema pallidum*. It is an extremely serious disease that, in the unlikely event that it is left untreated, can lead to sterility, damage to the central nervous system (CNS), and death. Approximately 3 weeks following infection, the patient may develop a primary syphilitic *chancre*, which is a

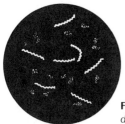

Figure 7-6. *Syphilis is the most dangerous of sexually transmitted diseases.*

painless ulcer with a clean base and a slightly elevated red rim. The chancre is found at the site of infection of the vulva, vagina, cervix, or penis. There may be swelling of lymph nodes in the groin. The presence of syphilis may be diagnosed through the finding of spirochetes on a dark-field microscopic examination of secretions taken from the chancre (Figure 7-6), or alternately by a blood test (serology). The treatment for primary syphilis is penicillin or erythromycin if the patient if allergic to penicillin. These may be given at the family planning clinic, or at the referral source if necessary.

The primary chancre of syphilis usually heals within 6 weeks, even if no treatment is given. Thereafter, within 1–6 months, the patient may develop a transient rash (lasting for several weeks), including lesions on the palms and soles, or there may be development of condylomata lata (broad-based warty growths usually found around the genitalia and anus). The individual may also notice a sore throat, fever, or loss of hair from the scalp. These symptoms of secondary syphilis usually last for 3–6 months. During this stage the disease is extremely contagious and requires immediate treatment with penicillin.

Lymphogranuloma Venereum

Lymphogranuloma venereum (LGV) is a sexually transmitted disease caused by chlamydia. Approximately 1–3 weeks after contact a small painful vessicle (fluid-filled blister) develops at the site of infection, followed by swelling of nearby lymph nodes. The infected lymph nodes break down, and chronic abscesses with open sores and lymphatic scarring may develop. This may lead to formation of tumorlike masses in the labia of females, and both sexes may have perirectal involvement with the formation of abscesses and narrowing of the rectum. Following infection with LGV there is an increased incidence of rectal malignancy.

The diagnosis of LGV is made by the Frei skin test or the LGV complement fixation blood test. The treatment for LGV is tetracycline or sulfa drugs. Any patient with suspected LGV will require a physician for evaluation, treatment, and long-term follow-up.

Granuloma Inguinale

Granuloma inguinale occurs most commonly among people who live in tropical areas and is caused by the bacterium *Donovania granulomatis*. The infection is thought to be sexually transmitted and is perhaps the only STD also associated with a lack of personal cleanliness. The incubation period varies from 1 to 12 weeks after exposure. First a papule (a firm bump) appears, followed by ulceration and elevated masses of granulated tissue. The lesions spread slowly, and over years there may be progressive development with extensive ulcerations and skin scarring in the genital area, lower abdomen, buttocks, and thighs.

The diagnosis of granuloma inguinale is made by demonstration of "Donovan bodies" in a tissue specimen taken from an involved area. The treatment is usually tetracycline or ampicillin.

Chancroid

The primary chancre of syphilis may be confused with *chancroid*, which is a bacterial disease caused by *Hemophilus ducrei*. The chancroid lesion is distinguished from a syphilitic chancre by the fact that it is a painful, ragged ulcer that exudes pus from the base. It develops within a week after infection, and there are often tender, swollen lymph nodes in the groin. The diagnosis of chancroid is made by finding the bacilli on a microscopic Gram stain and by performing a dark-field examination or serology to rule out syphilis. The recommended treatment for chancroid is erythromycin. An oral sulfa preparation or a cephalosporin may also be used.

OTHER COMMON
HEALTH PROBLEMS

While serving contraceptive clients, the health provider will encounter a number of common medical problems that are not gynecological or sexually transmitted. For some people, seeking assistance for family planning may be their only contact with a health service for many years. The family planning practitioner should be familiar with the signs and symptoms of these conditions and have established procedures for referring patients for appropriate treatment. This section cannot be a guide to general medicine, but some of those conditions with particular relevance to family planning are discussed.

Anemia

There are many types of anemia. Anemia is usually defined by a hemoglobin of less than 10 g/100 ml or a hematocrit of 30%, but the level of laboratory values at which anemia is considered significant will vary according to local clinical standards. Mild cases of iron deficiency anemia—the most common form—can be treated with dietary or vitamin supplementation. Severe anemias will require referral to a physician. Anemia found in an IUD user is of particular concern since a possibly increased menstrual flow can aggravate the condition.

Diabetes

Diabetes may be suspected if there is a history of weight loss, excessive eating and drinking, and excessive urination. A strong family history of diabetes, excessive obesity, a history of delivering large babies (greater than 4000 g), or frequent yeast infections may also be indicative of a client at risk. The diagnosis of diabetes requires laboratory evaluation of glucose tolerance. As a predisposing risk factor for cardiovascular disease, diabetes is a relative contraindication to the use of oral contraceptives. In addition, the provider should be aware that the use of oral contraceptives may reduce glucose tolerance and increase insulin requirements for diabetic patients. Prediabetic patients may develop symptoms of diabetes earlier on the pill than otherwise.

Hypertension

The definition of hypertension (high blood pressure) will vary according to what is considered "significant" in a given country or region. Generally, a blood pressure of 140/90 mm Hg or greater is indicative of hypertension requiring referral. Hypertension is a risk factor in the development of cardiovascular disease and is therefore a relative contraindication to pill use. Since oral contraceptive use can be associated with the development of hypertension in some women, the provider should check a pill user's blood pressure on a regular basis as part of standard follow-up procedures. Pill-associated hypertension occurs in a small percentage of users, is usually mild, and disappears after oral contraceptives are stopped.

Excessive Weight

Excessive obesity cannot be meaningfully quantified, since it depends on physical build, sex, race, and various cultural factors. However, excessive weight is a risk factor for cardiovascular disease and diabetes. Although weight *loss* is often a symptom of diabetes, obesity can contribute to the development of diabetes, particularly in prediabetic adults. Pill use in obese clients should be considered carefully, therefore. In addition, excessive obesity will probably prevent both laparoscopy and minilaparotomy from being performed on an outpatient basis for female sterilization. Referral of obese clients for evaluation and therapy can be an important contribution to that person's future health.

Nutritional Deficiencies

A wide range of nutritional disorders may be encountered by a family planning provider. Individuals may be seen with signs of malnutrition such as emaciation, edema (swelling), protruding abdomen, skin or gum inflammation (dermatitis, gingivitis), and so on. All clients will need nutritional evaluation and therapy. Lactating women are especially vulnerable to nutritional problems and will require particular attention. Children who accompany their parents to the family planning clinic may also be malnourished and should be treated with equal concern.

Hepatitis

The finding of an enlarged or tender liver, jaundice, loss of appetite, or a history of weight loss may be suggestive of hepatitis and require physician consultation. Acute hepatitis or severe chronic liver disease are absolute contraindications to the use of oral contraceptives.

Migraine Headaches

Identification of the causes and severity of headaches is extremely difficult (see page 52). A history of severe recurrent throbbing headaches, often associated with visual disturbance and/or nausea, is suggestive of migraine and is a relative contraindication to pill use. Any client with severe intractable headaches should have a neurological evaluation if possible.

Epilepsy

A family planning client may report a history of uncontrolled seizures. These individuals should be referred for an appropriate evaluation. Women choosing oral contraceptives should not start taking their pill until their condition has been fully diagnosed and adequately treated.

Goiter

An enlarged thyroid gland may be noted among family planning clients on examination, especially in areas where goiter is endemic. When these clients are referred for treatment, the provider should, as always, ascertain what contraceptive method is being used. Oral contraceptives are known to alter some thyroid function tests, making the interpretation of test findings more difficult among pill users.

Emotional Disturbance

Obvious emotional disorders may be noted by the health provider when interviewing prospective family planning clients. The provider can assist these clients by arranging for an evaluation by an appropriate psychologist or psychiatrist.

Sexual Concerns

The provision of family planning services quite naturally raises related sexual concerns for some clients. These concerns can be physiological, psychological, or both. They cover a broad range, from misunderstandings about the genitals and their sexual functioning to concerns about interpersonal relationships such as the extent of mutual attraction or the frequency of intercourse. The most serious are symptoms of sexual distress—impotence, dyspareunia, and several other conditions.

Since many health providers either do not have the training to deal with such concerns or do not feel comfortable with them, family planning professionals should be particularly attuned to sexuality issues. A family planning provider who is not trained to be a sexuality counselor should take primary responsibility to arrange for referral of the client to an appropriate resource—a counselor, psychologist, or psychiatrist. In making a referral for these sensitive problems, the provider should clearly explain to the client why it is necessary—because the provider is not personally comfortable with the issue, or because appropriate therapy requires more sophisticated skills.

Selected Readings

Anonymous: Chancroid. Lancet 2: 747, October 2, 1982

Anonymous: Chancroid. Morbidity and Mortality Weekly Report 31(14): 173, April 16, 1982

Anonymous: Genital herpes infection. Morbidity and Mortality Weekly Report 31(11): 137, March 26, 1982

Anonymous: Sexually transmitted diseases treatment guidelines 1982. Morbidity and Mortality Weekly Report 31(2S): 35S, August 20, 1982

Anonymous: Treatment of sexually transmitted diseases. The Medical Letter 24(605): 29, March 19, 1982

Arnoff MS: Teaching about the sexually transmitted diseases, in Rosenzweig N, Pearsall P (eds): Sex Education for the Health Professions. New York, Grune & Stratton, 1978

Bates B: A Guide to Physical Examination (ed 2). Philadephia, Lippincott Co, 1979

Benenson AS: Control of Communicable Diseases in Man (ed 12). Washington, DC, American Public Health Association, 1976

Fast MV, Nsanze H, D'Costa LJ, et al: Treatment of chancroid by clavulanic acid with amoxicilin in patients with beta-lactamase-positive *Hemophilus ducreyi* infection. Lancet 2: 509, September 4, 1982

Green R (ed): Human Sexuality: A Health Practitioner's Text. Baltimore, Williams & Wilkins, 1975

Harrison: Principles of Internal Medicine (ed 7). New York, McGraw-Hill, 1974

Hulka BS: Risk factors for cervical cancer. Journal of Chronic Diseases 35:3, 1982

Keith L, Brittain J: Sexually Transmitted Diseases. Aspen, Creative Informatics Inc, 1978

Kolodny R, et al: Textbook of Sexual Medicine. Boston, Little, Brown, 1979

McCormack WM: Sexually transmitted diseases: Women as victims. Journal of the American Medical Association 248(2): 177, July 9, 1982

McLellan R, Spence MR, Brockman M, et al: The clinical diagnosis of trichomoniasis. Obstetrics and Gynecology 60(1): 30, July 1982

Monif GRG: Obstetrical-Gynecological Infectious Diseases (ed 2). Gainesville, FL, Infectious Diseases Inc, 1981

Moore DE, Spadoni LR, Foy HM, et al: Increased frequency of serum antibodies to *Chlamydia trachomiatis* in infertility due to distal tubal disease. Lancet 2: 574, September 11, 1982

Sweet RL: Chlamydial salpingitis and infertility. Fertility and Sterility 38(5): 530, November 1982

Index